Arthritis Relief

Arthritis Relief

氣功防治關節炎

Chinese Qigong for
Healing and Prevention

Dr. Yang, Jwing-Ming

YMAA Publication Center
Wolfeboro, NH USA

YMAA Publication Center, Inc.
Main Office
PO Box 480
Wolfeboro, NH
038941-800-669-8892 • www.ymaa.com • info@ymaa.com

Editor: James O'Leary
Cover Design: Katya Popova

ISBN-10: 1-59439-033-9
ISBN-13: 978-1-59439-033-3

20200304

Publisher's Cataloging in Publication

Yang, Jwing Ming, 1946-

Arthritis relief : Chinese qigong for healing and prevention / Yang, Jwing-Ming. -- 3rd ed. -- Boston, Mass. : YMAA Publication Center, 2005.

p. ; cm.

Second ed. published as: Arthritis : the Chinese way of healing and prevention.
Includes bibliographical references and index.
ISBN: 1-59439-033-9
ISBN 13: 978-1-59439-033-3

1. Arthritis--Alternative treatment. 2. Qi gong. 3. Medicine, Chinese. I. Title. II. Chinese qigong for healing and prevention.

RC933 .Y36 2005   2005925610
616.7/2206--dc22   0506

Disclaimer:
The author and publisher of this material are NOT RESPONSIBLE in any manner whatsoever for any injury which may occur through reading or following the instructions in this manual.
The activities, physical or otherwise, described in this material may be too strenuous or dangerous for some people, and the reader(s) should consult a physician before engaging in them.

Figures 1-15 and 1-16 from the *LifeART Collection of Images* ©1989-1997 by Techpool Studios, Columbus, OH.

Printed in USA

Dedicated to My Mother
Madame Yang, Xie-Jin
楊謝盡女士

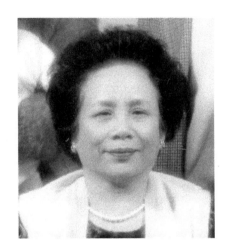

Contents

About the Author

Dr. Yang, Jwing-Ming, Ph.D. 楊俊敏博士

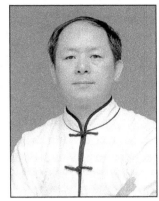

Dr. Yang, Jwing-Ming was born on August 11th, 1946, in Xinzhu Xian (新竹縣), Taiwan (台灣), Republic of China (中華民國). He started his Wushu (武術) (Gongfu or Kung Fu, 功夫) training at the age of fifteen under the Shaolin White Crane (Bai He, 少林白鶴) Master Cheng, Gin-Gsao (曾金灶) (1911-1976). Master Cheng originally learned Taizuquan (太祖拳) from his grandfather when he was a child. When Master Cheng was fifteen years old, he started learning White Crane from Master Jin, Shao-Feng (金紹峰), and followed him for twenty-three years until Master Jin's death.

In thirteen years of study (1961-1974) under Master Cheng, Dr. Yang became an expert in the White Crane Style of Chinese martial arts, which includes both the use of barehands and of various weapons such as saber, staff, spear, trident, two short rods, and many other weapons. With the same master he also studied White Crane Qigong (氣功), Qin Na (or Chin Na, 擒拿), Tui Na (推拿) and Dian Xue massages (點穴按摩), and herbal treatment.

At the age of sixteen, Dr. Yang began the study of Yang Style Taijiquan (楊氏太極拳) under Master Gao, Tao (高濤). After learning from Master Gao, Dr. Yang continued his study and research of Taijiquan with several masters and senior practitioners such as Master Li, Mao-Ching (李茂清) and Mr. Wilson Chen (陳威伸) in Taipei (台北). Master Li learned his Taijiquan from the well-known Master Han, Ching-Tang (韓慶堂), and Mr. Chen learned his Taijiquan from Master Zhang, Xiang-San (張祥三). Dr. Yang has mastered the Taiji barehand sequence, pushing hands, the two-man fighting sequence, Taiji sword, Taiji saber, and Taiji Qigong.

When Dr. Yang was eighteen years old he entered Tamkang College (淡江學院) in Taipei Xian (台北縣) to study Physics. In college he began the study of traditional Shaolin Long Fist (Changquan or Chang Chuan, 少林長拳) with Master Li, Mao-Ching at the Tamkang College Guoshu Club (淡江國術社) (1964-1968), and eventually became an assistant instructor under Master Li. In 1971 he completed his M.S. degree in Physics at the National Taiwan University (台灣大學), and then served in the Chinese Air Force from 1971 to 1972. In the service, Dr. Yang taught Physics at the Junior Academy of the Chinese Air Force (空軍幼校) while also teaching Wushu. After being honorably discharged in 1972, he returned to Tamkang College to teach Physics and resumed study under Master Li, Mao-Ching. From Master Li, Dr. Yang learned Northern Style Wushu, which includes both barehand (especially kicking) techniques and numerous weapons.

In 1974, Dr. Yang came to the United States to study Mechanical Engineering at Purdue University. At the request of a few students, Dr. Yang began to teach Gongfu

(Kung Fu), which resulted in the foundation of the Purdue University Chinese Kung Fu Research Club in the spring of 1975. While at Purdue, Dr. Yang also taught college-credited courses in Taijiquan. In May of 1978 he was awarded a Ph.D. in Mechanical Engineering by Purdue.

In 1980, Dr. Yang moved to Houston to work for Texas Instruments. While in Houston he founded Yang's Shaolin Kung Fu Academy, which was eventually taken over by his disciple Mr. Jeffery Bolt after moving to Boston in 1982. Dr. Yang founded Yang's Martial Arts Academy (YMAA) in Boston on October 1, 1982.

In January of 1984 he gave up his engineering career to devote more time to research, writing, and teaching. In March of 1986 he purchased property in the Jamaica Plain area of Boston to be used as the headquarters of the new organization, Yang's Martial Arts Association (YMAA). The organization has continued to expand, and, as of July 1st 1989, YMAA has become just one division of Yang's Oriental Arts Association, Inc. (YOAA, Inc.).

In summary, Dr. Yang has been involved in Chinese Wushu since 1961. During this time, he has spent thirteen years learning Shaolin White Crane (Bai He), Shaolin Long Fist (Changquan), and Taijiquan. Dr. Yang has more than thirty-three years of instructional experience: seven years in Taiwan, five years at Purdue University, two years in Houston, Texas, and nineteen years in Boston, Massachusetts.

In addition, Dr. Yang has also been invited to offer seminars around the world to share his knowledge of Chinese martial arts and Qigong. The countries he has visited include Argentina, Austria, Barbados, Botswana, Belgium, Bermuda, Canada, Chile, England, France, Germany, Holland, Hungary, Ireland, Italy, Latvia, Mexico, Poland, Portugal, Saudi Arabia, Spain, South Africa, Switzerland, and Venezuela.

Since 1986, YMAA has become an international organization, which currently includes 56 schools located in Argentina, Belgium, Canada, Chile, France, Holland, Hungary, Iran, Ireland, Italy, Poland, Portugal, South Africa, United Kingdom, Venezuela, and the United States. Many of Dr. Yang's books and videotapes have been translated into languages such as French, Italian, Spanish, Polish, Czech, Bulgarian, Russian, Hungarian, and Iranian.

Dr. Yang has published thirty-one other volumes on the martial arts and Qigong:

1. *Shaolin Chin Na*; Unique Publications, Inc., 1980.

2. *Shaolin Long Fist Kung Fu*; Unique Publications, Inc., 1981.

3. *Yang Style Tai Chi Chuan*; Unique Publications, Inc., 1981.

4. *Introduction to Ancient Chinese Weapons*; Unique Publications, Inc., 1985.

5. *Qigong for Health and Martial Arts*; YMAA Publication Center, 1985.

6. *Northern Shaolin Sword*; YMAA Publication Center, 1985.

7. *Tai Chi Theory and Martial Power*; YMAA Publication Center, 1986.

8. *Tai Chi Chuan Martial Applications*, YMAA Publication Center, 1986.

9. *Analysis of Shaolin Chin Na*; YMAA Publication Center, 1987.

10. *Eight Simple Qigong Exercises for Health*; YMAA Publication Center, 1988.

11. *The Root of Chinese Qigong—The Secrets of Qigong Training*; YMAA Publication Center, 1989.

12. *Qigong—The Secret of Youth*; YMAA Publication Center, 1989.

13. *Xingyiquan—Theory and Applications*; YMAA Publication Center, 1990.

14. *The Essence of Taiji Qigong—Health and Martial Arts*; YMAA Publication Center, 1990.

15. *Qigong for Arthritis*; YMAA Publication Center, 1991(this volume).

16. *Chinese Qigong Massage—General Massage*; YMAA Publication Center, 1992.

17. *How to Defend Yourself*; YMAA Publication Center, 1992.

18. *Baguazhang—Emei Baguazhang*; YMAA Publication Center, 1994.

19. *Comprehensive Applications of Shaolin Chin Na—The Practical Defense of Chinese Seizing Arts*; YMAA Publication Center, 1995.

20. *Taiji Chin Na—The Seizing Art of Taijiquan*; YMAA Publication Center, 1995.

21. *The Essence of Shaolin White Crane*; YMAA Publication Center, 1996.

22. *Back Pain—Chinese Qigong for Healing and Prevention*; YMAA Publication Center, 1997 (2nd edition 2004);

23. *Ancient Chinese Weapons*; YMAA Publication Center, 1999.

24. *Taijiquan—Classical Yang Style*; YMAA Publication Center, 1999.

25. *Tai Chi Secrets of Ancient Masters*; YMAA Publication Center, 1999.

26. *Taiji Sword—Classical Yang Style*; YMAA Publication Center, 1999.

27. *Tai Chi Secrets of Wu and Li Styles*; YMAA Publication Center, 2001.

28. *Tai Chi Secrets of Yang Style*; YMAA Publication Center, 2001.

29. *Tai Chi Secrets of Wu Style*; YMAA Publication Center, 2002.

30. *Taijiquan Theory of Dr. Yang, Jwing-Ming*; YMAA Publication Center, 2003.

31. *Qigong Meditation—Embryonic Breathing*; YMAA Publication Center, 2003.

32. *Qigong Meditation—Small Circulation*; YMAA Publication Center, 2005.

Dr. Yang has also published the following videotapes and DVD:

Videotapes:

1. *Yang Style Tai Chi Chuan and Its Applications*; YMAA Publication Center, 1984.

2. *Shaolin Long Fist Kung Fu—Lien Bu Chuan and Its Applications*; YMAA Publication Center, 1985.

3. *Shaolin Long Fist Kung Fu—Gung Li Chuan and Its Applications*; YMAA Publication Center, 1986.

4. *Shaolin Chin Na*; YMAA Publication Center, 1987.

5. *Eight Simple Qigong Exercises—The Eight Pieces of Brocade*; YMAA Publication Center, 1987, 2003.

6. *The Essence of Taiji Qigong*; YMAA Publication Center, 1990.

7. *Qigong for Arthritis*; YMAA Publication Center, 1991.

8. *Qigong Massage—Self Massage*; YMAA Publication Center, 1992.

9. *Qigong Massage—With a Partner*; YMAA Publication Center, 1992.

10. *Defend Yourself 1—Unarmed Attack*; YMAA Publication Center, 1992.

11. *Defend Yourself 2—Knife Attack*; YMAA Publication Center, 1992.

12. *Comprehensive Applications of Shaolin Chin Na 1*; YMAA Publication Center, 1995.

13. *Comprehensive Applications of Shaolin Chin Na 2*; YMAA Publication Center, 1995.

14. *Shaolin Long Fist Kung Fu—Yi Lu Mai Fu & Er Lu Mai Fu*; YMAA Publication Center, 1995.

15. *Shaolin Long Fist Kung Fu—Shi Zi Tang*; YMAA Publication Center, 1995.

16. Taiji Chin Na; YMAA Publication Center, 1995.

17. *Emei Baguazhang—1; Basic Training, Qigong, Eight Palms, and Applications*; YMAA Publication Center, 1995.

18. *Emei Baguazhang—2; Swimming Body Baguazhang and Its Applications*; YMAA Publication Center, 1995.

19. *Emei Baguazhang—3; Bagua Deer Hook Sword and Its Applications*; YMAA Publication Center, 1995.

20. *Xingyiquan—12 Animal Patterns and Their Applications*; YMAA Publication Center, 1995.

21. *24 and 48 Simplified Taijiquan*; YMAA Publication Center, 1995.

22. *White Crane Hard Qigong*; YMAA Publication Center, 1997.

23. *White Crane Soft Qigong*; YMAA Publication Center, 1997.

24. *Xiao Hu Yan—Intermediate Level Long Fist Sequence*; YMAA Publication Center, 1997.

25. *Back Pain—Chinese Qigong for Healing and Prevention*; YMAA Publication Center, 1997.

26. *Scientific Foundation of Chinese Qigong*; YMAA Publication Center, 1997.

27. *Taijiquan—Classical Yang Style*; YMAA Publication Center, 1999.

28. *Taiji Sword—Classical Yang Style*; YMAA Publication Center, 1999.

29. *Chin Na in Depth—1*; YMAA Publication Center, 2000.

30. *Chin Na in Depth—2*; YMAA Publication Center, 2000.

31. *San Cai Jian & Its Applications*; YMAA Publication Center, 2000.

32. *Kun Wu Jian & Its Applications*; YMAA Publication Center, 2000.

33. *Qi Men Jian & Its Applications*; YMAA Publication Center, 2000.

34. *Chin Na in Depth—3*; YMAA Publication Center, 2001.

35. *Chin Na in Depth—4*; YMAA Publication Center, 2001.

36. *Chin Na in Depth—5*; YMAA Publication Center, 2001.

37. *Chin Na in Depth—6*; YMAA Publication Center, 2001.

38. *12 Routines Tan Tui*; YMAA Publication Center, 2001.

39. *Chin Na in Depth—7*; YMAA Publication Center, 2002.

40. *Chin Na in Depth—8*; YMAA Publication Center, 2002.

41. *Chin Na in Depth—9*; YMAA Publication Center, 2002.

42. *Chin Na in Depth—10*; YMAA Publication Center, 2002.

43. *Chin Na in Depth—11*; YMAA Publication Center, 2002.

44. *Chin Na in Depth—12*; YMAA Publication Center, 2002.

45. *White Crane Gongfu—1*; YMAA Publication Center, 2002.

46. *White Crane Gongfu—2*; YMAA Publication Center, 2002.

47. *Taijiquan Pushing Hands—1*; YMAA Publication Center, 2003.

48. *Taijiquan Pushing Hands—2*; YMAA Publication Center, 2003.

49. *Taiji Saber and Its Applications*; YMAA Publication Center, 2003.

50. *Taiji Symbol Sticking Hands—1*; YMAA Publication Center, 2003.

51. *Taiji Ball Qigong—1*; YMAA Publication Center, 2003.

52. *Taiji Ball Qigong—2*; YMAA Publication Center, 2003.

53. *Taiji Ball Qigong—3*; YMAA Publication Center, 2004.

54. *Taiji Ball Qigong—4*; YMAA Publication Center, 2004.

55. *Taijiquan Pushing Hands—3*; YMAA Publication Center, 2004.

56. *Taijiquan Pushing Hands—4*; YMAA Publication Center, 2004.

57. *Shaolin Kung Fu—1*; YMAA Publication Center, 2004.

58. *Shaolin Kung Fu—2*; YMAA Publication Center, 2004.

59. *Taiji & Shaolin Staff Fundamental Training—1*; YMAA Publication Center, 2004.

60. *Advanced Practical Chin Na—1*; YMAA Publication Center, 2004.

61. *Advanced Practical Chin Na—2*; YMAA Publication Center, 2004.

62. *Taiji Chin Na In-Depth—1*; YMAA Publication Center, 2004.

63. *Taiji Chin Na In-Depth—2*; YMAA Publication Center, 2004.

64. *Taiji Chin Na In-Depth—3*; YMAA Publication Center, 2004.

65. *Taiji Chin Na In-Depth—4*; YMAA Publication Center, 2004.

66. *Tai Chi Fighting Set*; YMAA Publication Center, 2004.

DVDs:

1. *Chin Na in Depth—1, 2, 3, 4*; YMAA Publication Center, 2003.

2. *White Crane Qigong*; YMAA Publication Center, 2003.

3. *Taijiquan, Classical Yang Style*; YMAA Publication Center, 2003.

4. *Chin Na in Depth—5, 6, 7, 8*; YMAA Publication Center, 2003.

5. *Chin Na in Depth—9, 10, 11, 12*; YMAA Publication Center, 2003.

6. *Eight Simple Qigong Exercises for Health*, YMAA Publication Center, 2003.

7. *Shaolin White Crane Gong Fu—Basic Training, 1 & 2*; YMAA Publication Center, 2004.

8. *Analysis of Shaolin Chin Na*; YMAA Publication Center, 2004.

Foreword (from the First Edition)

Dr. Thomas G. Gutheil, M.D.
Associate Professor of Psychiatry,
Harvard Medical School

The book you are about to read further illuminates the application of ancient Chinese teachings and practices to contemporary health problems and extends the valuable contributions of Dr. Yang, Jwing-Ming to the task of enabling Western readers to discover important long-unavailable Eastern texts.

The potentially beneficial expansion of the total repertoire of health information, by such addition of Oriental teachings on health and disease, has, regrettably, met with occasional ill-advised but powerful resistance. In September of 1990, Newsweek magazine carried a story under the heading "Medicine" which was entitled, "Does Doctor Know Best?" *Newsweek* told the following story.

A 39 year-old Chinese woman named Julia Cheng, living in Connecticut, had a daughter named Shirley who had suffered since the age of 11 months from a severe and crippling childhood disease, Juvenile Rheumatoid Arthritis. As a woman from two cultures, Mrs. Cheng had had her daughter's illness treated in both America and mainland China. American specialists tended to use standard medications in the treatment of this crippling disease; physicians in China offered a combination of herbal and physical therapies. While the evidence from the child's own history seemed to indicate that a blend of Western and Chinese therapies brought some relief for the child's condition, her deterioration continued relentlessly, so that at the age of 7 (at the time the article was written), the child was in constant pain, and confined to a wheelchair.

During the Chinese revolutionary period, the mother's trip could not take place, so that she had to seek help from a local physician. The child's Connecticut physician recommended surgical repair of the child's knees, hips, and left ankle. The child's mother, by all evidence, presumably competent to make this decision, rejected this recommended operation and expressed her intentions to take the child to China (when that was safe) for less extensive surgery combined with traditional Chinese treatments (recall that Western-Eastern combined therapy had had some success before). However, the mother's refusal of the proposed operation triggered various child-protective actions by Connecticut's Department of Child and Youth Services, following guidelines in the laws designed to cover children thought to be at risk for parental neglect. Thus, the child was taken into custody by the public agency, and a superior court judge authorized the operation. For a physician in my field—forensic psychiatry and medical legal topics in general—this case has many interesting features in several realms: the question of informed consent to medical treatment; the right of competent individuals to reject treatment (even, theoretically, life saving treatments); problems of cross-cultural issues in individuals who are making complex health-care decisions; racism and sexism in American medical and legal practice (as might relate to the fact that the patient was both a woman and Chinese); and many other clinical, legal and ethical questions. What I want to bring out here, however, and what leads me to begin my foreword to this book with this case, is that it reveals the perception, at least by our judicial system, and almost certainly of the American medical system, that Western and Oriental approaches in a real life case of arthritis were simply not reconcilable.

Note that Mrs. Cheng was not planning to give her child no treatment (i.e., to deprive the child of treatment); nor to give the child some idiosyncratic treatment (such as laetrile for cancer); nor to use non-medical religious methods of healing, as in some of the Christian Science legal cases that have been much in the news lately Instead, Mrs. Cheng was planning to procure an active treatment regimen for her child, a regimen which drew upon a history of medical research, diagnosis, and treatment extending back for literally thousands of years; and which, more importantly, had been empirically demonstrated to have some beneficial effects in this child specifically.

Understanding the regrettable case described above may have one indirect beneficial effect: it illuminates an inherent strength of the present volume. This volume makes as close a study as exists today of the application of ancient Chinese principles regarding Qi to the troubling condition of arthritis. Since many of the source texts for this study were only recently available, much less translated, this book makes it possible, for the first time, for Western readers to expand the repertoire of treatments for one of the most disabling of all diseases, by adding to any Western regimen this time-tested and systematic approach. Drawing heavily upon mental and emotional states, thought and mind, mood and morale, as well as upon what would now be described in Western terms as "low impact exercises," this text provides, to Western readers and sufferers of arthritis alike, an innovative and immensely valuable complement to the therapeutic armamentarium.

We must applaud Dr. Yang's efforts to make not only available, but also accessible and comprehensible, these ancient principles. While this volume fits best into the sequence of explorations listed elsewhere in this book, it is designed to stand on its own and to provide summary reviews of the basic ideas which it attempts to synthesize. The interested reader is in for a remarkably clear and organized discussion of a neglected subject area whose sufferers are legion.

Foreword (for the New Edition)

Perry A. Chapdelaine, Sr.
Author and Executive Director,
The Arthritis Fund

Until the exceptional journey of Marco Polo in the thirteenth century, Europeans viewed scientific, religious, medical, and philosophical ideas in a very limited manner, perceiving themselves as the world's, if not the universe's center.

Marco Polo brought to Western consciousness but a tiny fraction of long-accumulated Chinese wisdom, including knowledge of the invention of gun powder, the printing press, rocketry, and of course, the shocking revelation of a huge civilization already thousands of years old.

Had leaders of thirteenth century Western thought been sufficiently open to new ideas, Marco Polo could have prepared us for a workable medical system based on the Chinese concept of primary energy, a subtle bioelectric force pervading our every cell, common to us all, and capable of preventing illness, healing when ill, and extending life and its quality.

While a great deal of Chinese wisdom was still locked up in the archives of special teachers (masters) under the seal of secrecy, we would nonetheless have learned much about healing from the vast array of material already available in the thirteenth century; acupuncture, herbology, massage, beneficial breathing techniques, and most importantly, the many ways to manipulate and to increase the flow of this subtle energy force called Qi (pronounced Chee).

Apparently, Western consciousness is at last prepared to receive this grand Chinese legacy, because Qigong (energy work) knowledge and training have proliferated in Western society in the last twenty years. Western medicine has begun to accept, or at least explore, the existence of Qi and its circulation in the body.

Yang, Jwing-Ming, Ph.D. is indeed a master when describing in numerous published volumes the extensive Chinese concept of Qi, explaining not just well-known facets of the lore, but also revealing long-hidden secret manuscripts previously unavailable to Western readers.

Dr. Yang's *Arthritis Relief—Chinese Qigong for Healing and Prevention* describes how virtually all disease states, including the many forms of arthritis, can be conquered or changed by deliberately influencing our own store and flow of bioelectric current.

With the guidance of Dr. Yang, the reader will learn many simple exercises which condition the tissues and permit increased blood flow, and thus oxygen and other nourishment, to those parts of the body in need.

More importantly, the reader is taught to "lead" the Qi to direct the flow of this primary subtle energy, According to Dr. Yang, "In order to use Qigong to maintain and improve your health you must know that there is Qi in your body, and you must understand how it circulates and what you can do to insure that the circulation is smooth and strong." All this, and more, is presented in clear language that flows easily from a very patient teacher.

As a representative of a non-profit, charity foundation dedicated to wiping the scourge of arthritis from the earth's face, and because of the quality and content of Arthritis Relief—Chinese Qigong for Healing and Prevention, my Board of Directors could do no less than prompt me to recommend this book to the millions of Americans who suffer from the various forms of this disease. Four thousand years of Chinese observation has resulted in many beneficial methods for preventing illness and achieving wellness, and none are more basic to the arthritic than those described in this book.

Preface (First Edition)

Arthritis has afflicted humankind for as far back as we can trace. In all races, the young as well as the old have experienced the pain of arthritis. The condition can also have a disastrous effect on the sufferer's peace of mind. Despite the great advances made in many fields of science, Western medicine today is still unable to cure many forms of arthritis. Most treatment is limited to relieving pain and inflammation, rather than curing the condition at its root.

In the nearly four thousand years that Chinese medicine has been developing, many approaches have emerged to stopping the pain or even curing arthritis, such as acupuncture, massage, Qigong (氣功) (pronounced "Chee Gong") exercises, and herbal treatment.

Naturally, some methods are more effective than others, depending on the condition of the specific individual. Qigong exercises have come to be considered as an excellent method not only of preventing arthritis, but also of curing many forms of arthritis and in rebuilding the strength of the joints. Once the joint completely recovers its strength, it is well on its way to a complete healing.

In all of human history, now is the first opportunity that all of the world's cultures have had to get to know each other; we would be foolish to pass up this opportunity to learn from each other. It is clear that both Western and Oriental medicines have their advantages and disadvantages. For example, Western medicine has traditionally ignored the existence of the energy (Qi or bioelectricity) part of the body and has paid more attention to the body's physical problems. Chinese medicine, on the other hand, has traditionally paid more attention to the empirical development of treatments and has ignored scientific research aimed at developing the theoretical background and more advanced equipment for both diagnosis and treatment.

If both cultures can share what they have discovered and learn to experience each other with open minds, then medicine would have a chance to begin a new era. Western medicine, for example, would be able to borrow the information which Chinese medicine has accumulated about Qi (氣) (bioelectricity) and combine it with the findings drawn from its own experience. Chinese medicine, on the other hand, could adapt modern Western medical technology to aid and improve the effectiveness of traditional Oriental medicine.

Arthritis serves as an excellent demonstration of how this combination of Eastern and Western medicine can work. Chinese doctors believe that the main causes of arthritis are weakness and injury of the joints. In order to rebuild the strength of the joints and repair the injury, Qi must be led to these joints and must be able to circulate smoothly there. Only by nourishing these joints with Qi can the damage be repaired. Chinese doctors have researched ways of improving the Qi circulation in the joints, and have found that the majority of arthritis patients can be healed. In addition, they have found that, once the joints are strong again, the arthritis will not readily return.

Chinese Qigong (energy work) improves the Qi circulation through both mental and physical training. In this book I will focus only on the Qigong practices commonly used by the Chinese to treat arthritis. Other methods, such as acupuncture and herbal treatments, will have to be introduced elsewhere by qualified Chinese physicians. I hope that this book will help many Western arthritis sufferers regain their health.

The first chapter in this book will briefly discuss the general concepts of Chinese Qigong; the second chapter will summarize some information about arthritis. The third chapter will explain the theory of how Qigong cures arthritis; and finally, the fourth chapter will present some Qigong exercises for arthritis.

In order to be consistent with international usage, we have decided that in this book we will begin to use the Pinyin system for spelling of Chinese words. We hope that this will be more convenient for those readers who consult other Chinese books. However, in order to avoid confusion, commonly accepted spellings of names will not be changed, such as Tamkang College and Taipei.

Preface (New Edition)

Since the first edition of this book was published, numerous people have contacted both me and the YMAA Publications Center about the benefits they have obtained from this book. Many of them could not believe that the serious problem of arthritis can be easily treated by simple relaxed exercises. Through acupuncture, massage, or herbal treatment, the relief from arthritis pain is not as long lasting, yet is also drug free and promotes a healthier lifestyle. It is also well understood that the long-term solution is through the correct methods of exercises. For example, when an episode is serious, any exercise that can cause tension in the joint area is not proper. This is because the tension of the joint locks the joint, making the Qi and blood circulation more stagnant. The key to healing or repairing the joints is through adequate, smooth Qi and blood circulation. Only then the damaged physical areas be rebuilt.

I remember when I was teaching Qigong in Andover, Massachusetts about ten years ago, right after my class, there was a senior woman who came to see me for help. She showed me her swollen hands and wrists, caused from a serious arthritis problem. After I took a look, I asked her if she was able to move her fingers and turn her wrists. She tried and showed some capability of moving them with limited flexibility. I taught her some simple theory of the importance of circulating the Qi and blood in the fingers and wrists. Then, I encouraged her to do the finger and wrist exercises everyday as many times as possible. I also told her it would probably take six months to see the effectiveness of the treatment.

Three months later, she came to see me although I had forgotten about our first meeting and conversation. She showed me her hands, and what I saw were mildly swollen index, middle, and ring fingers. I told her she should be careful, since there was a sign of arthritis development. She stared at me with big eyes and said: "You don't member me, Dr. Yang" and she refreshed my memory of the first meeting. I could not believe it took only three months for her to have this significant progress. She told me she had stopped taking pain killer for nearly a month already. Whenever there was an episode of pain, she simply moved the area for a few minutes and the pain alleviated.

From this experience, I had seen how she had conquered herself in making these activities part of her lifestyle. I also believe that she had grasped the key to healing herself through simple Qigong exercises.

Many people think Qigong practice is hard and mysterious. In some ways, it is. However, in some other ways, it is simple and effective. Actually, the most difficult task is regulating yourself into practicing as part of your lifestyle. Remember, the most powerful way to maintain health and curing problems is to bring some proper daily exercises and diet into your life. Our physical body is evolved through use and movement. We must keep moving and exercising it. If we ignore this fact, we will degenerate rapidly and become sick easily.

Dr. Yang, Jwing-Ming
Naples , Italy
March 26, 2004

Romanization of Chinese Words

This book uses the Pinyin romanization system of Chinese to English. Pinyin is standard in the People's Republic of China, and in several world organizations, including the United Nations. Pinyin, which was introduced in China in the 1950's, replaces the Wade-Giles and Yale systems. In some cases, the more popular spelling of a word may be used for clarity.

Some common conversions:

Pinyin	Also Spelled As	Pronunciation
Qi	Chi	chē
Qigong	Chi Kung	chē kŭng
Qin Na	Chin Na	chǐn nǎ
Jin	Jing	jǐn
Gongfu	Kung Fu	gŏng foo
Taijiquan	Tai Chi Chuan	tī jē chüén

For more information, please refer to *The People's Republic of China: Administrative Atlas, The Reform of the Chinese Written Language,* or a contemporary manual of style.

The author and publisher have taken the liberty of not italicizing words of foreign origin in this text. This decision was made to make the text easier to read. Please see the comprehensive glossary for definitions of Chinese words.

Acknowledgments (First Edition)

Thanks to A. Reza Farman-Farmaian for the photography and Wen-Ching Wu for the drawings. Thanks also to David Ripianzi, James O'Leary, Jr. Jeffrey Pratt, Jenifer Menefee and many other YMAA members for proofing the manuscript and for contributing many valuable suggestions and discussions. Special thanks to Alan Dougall for his editing; and deepest appreciation to Dr. Thomas Gutheil for his continued support.

Acknowledgments (New Edition)

Thanks to Tim Comrie for his typesetting. Thanks to Erik Elsemans, Ciaran Harris, and Susan Bullowa for proofing the manuscript and contributing many valuable suggestions and discussions. Special thanks to Katya Popova for the cover design, to James O'Leary for editing. Also, special thanks to Dr. Thomas G. Gutheil for his continued support.

CHAPTER 1

About Chinese Qigong
中國氣功介紹

1-1. INTRODUCTION 介紹

Young and old, rich and poor, all have experienced the pain of arthritis. Because it is so prevalent, almost all cultures have developed ways of alleviating the pain or even curing the condition.

Generally speaking, younger people get arthritis less frequently than the elderly because their bodies are in better condition, and they are more active. Experience has also shown that, once younger people do develop arthritis, they recover more easily. Poor people have tended to get arthritis less frequently than wealthier people, because they engage in more manual labor. This seems to indicate that people who exercise regularly have a better chance of staying healthy and free from arthritis.

As in other cultures, the Chinese also suffer both physically and mentally from arthritis. Many methods of healing and prevention have been developed within the tradition of Chinese medicine.

The most fundamental principle of Chinese medicine is the concept of Qi (氣) (pronounced "Chee," known today in the West as bioelectricity). Illnesses are diagnosed by evaluating the condition of the body's Qi and interpreting the visible physical symptoms. According to Chinese medicine, when the Qi and its supply start to become unbalanced, the physical body is affected and begins to be damaged. This can happen both if the body is too Yin (陰) (deficient in Qi) or too Yang (陽) (with an excess of Qi). When Chinese physicians diagnose any disease or condition, they explore how and where the Qi is unbalanced. Once the Qi imbalance is corrected and the Qi returned to its normal level, the root cause of the illness has been removed.

Acupuncture is a common method for adjusting the Qi and preventing further physical damage. The Qi level can also be raised or lowered to stimulate the repair of the damage.

Applying Qi theory to arthritis can clear up many mysteries that cannot be explained by Western medicine. For example, almost all Western studies have denied that arthritis is significantly affected by the weather, despite the insistence of many arthritis sufferers. However, if we accept the fact that our bodies have a bioelectric field, it should be obvious that it would be affected by a strong natural electric field such as that found in thunderclouds. In fact, this external natural electric field can also disturb our emotions, because they are also affected by Qi imbalances in our body. The West has recently discovered that our internal bioelectric field can be disturbed by the electromagnetic field generated by high tension wires, and that this may cause cancer.

In China, acupuncture is not the only method used to correct the Qi imbalance that causes arthritis. Massage, cavity press (acupressure), and certain Qigong (氣功) (pronounced "Chee Gong") exercises are also used. Most of these methods were created by medical doctors, but some were also created by masters of the Qigong systems used by martial artists. This is not as odd as it would at first seem. Since joint injuries are common among martial artists, many of these injuries would have developed into arthritis, a dangerous condition in a time when martial arts were used in deadly earnest. Many of the masters were experienced in Qigong and in elements of medicine, especially in the treatment of injuries, much like our modern sports medicine specialists. It would therefore be natural for them to find ways treat a common condition like arthritis. Most people in the West are familiar with the slow, relaxed movements of Taijiquan (太極拳) (or Tai Chi Chuan). In China, this art is well known for its ability to rebuild the strength of the joints and alleviate the causes of arthritis.

While Western medicine has developed according to the principle of diagnosing visible symptoms and curing visible physical damage, Chinese medicine may be more advanced in that it deals with the body's Qi. On the other hand, Chinese medicine is still far behind Western medicine in the study of and research on the physical aspect of the human body. This can be seen in Western scientific methods and in the technology the West has developed. Because of the differences between the two systems of medicine, there are still large gaps in mankind's understanding of the body. I believe that if both medical cultures can learn and borrow from each other, these remaining gaps can soon be filled, and medicine as a whole will be able to take a giant step forward.

The ease of communication and the increased friendship among many different cultures during the last two decades has given mankind an unprecedented opportunity to share such things as medical concepts. We should all take advantage of this and open our minds to the knowledge and experiences of other peoples. I sincerely hope that this takes place, especially in the field of medicine. This goal has been my motivation in writing this book. Because of my limited knowledge, I can only offer this little volume. I hope that it generates widening ripples of interest in sharing and exchanging with other cultures.

1-2. Qi, Qigong, and Man 氣、氣功與人之關係

Before we discuss the relationship of Qi to the human body, we should first define Qi and Qigong. We will first discuss the general concept of Qi, including both the traditional understanding and the possible modern scientific paradigms, which allows us to use modern concepts to explain Qigong. If you would like to investigate these subjects in more detail, please refer to the YMAA book: *The Root of Chinese Qigong*.

A General Definition of Qi 氣的廣義

Qi is the energy or natural force that fills the universe. The Chinese have traditionally believed that there are three major powers in the universe. These Three Powers (San Cai, 三才) are Heaven (Tian, 天), Earth (Di, 地), and Man (Ren, 人) (alternatively translated as "Humanity"). Heaven (the sky or universe) has Heaven Qi (Tian Qi), the most important of the three, that is made up of the forces which the heavenly bodies exert on the earth, such as sunshine, moonlight, gravity, and the energy from the stars. In ancient times, the Chinese believed that weather, climate, and natural disasters were governed by Heaven Qi. Chinese people still refer to the weather as Heaven Qi (Tian Qi, 天氣). Every energy field strives to stay in balance, so whenever the Heaven Qi loses its balance, it tries to rebalance itself. Then the wind must blow, rain must fall, even tornadoes or hurricanes must happen in order for the Heaven Qi to reach a new energy balance.

Under Heaven Qi, is Earth Qi (Di Qi, 地氣). It is influenced and controlled by Heaven Qi. For example, too much rain will force a river to flood or change its path. Without rain, the plants will die. The Chinese believe that Earth Qi is made up of lines and patterns of energy, as well as the earth's magnetic field and the heat concealed underground. These energies must also balance, otherwise disasters such as earthquakes will occur. When the Qi of the earth is balanced, plants will grow and animals thrive.

Finally, within the Earth Qi, each individual person, animal, and plant has its own Qi field, which always seeks to be balanced. When any individual being loses its Qi balance, it will sicken, die, and decompose. All natural things, including mankind and our Human Qi, grow within and are influenced by the natural cycles of Heaven Qi and Earth Qi. Throughout the history of Qigong, people have been most interested in Human Qi (Ren Qi, 人氣) and its relationship with Heaven Qi and Earth Qi.

In China, Qi is defined as any type of energy that is able to demonstrate power and strength. This energy can be electricity, magnetic, heat, or light. For examples, electric power is called "Electric Qi" (Dian Qi, 電氣), and heat is called "Heat Qi" (Re Qi, 熱氣). When a person is alive, his body's energy is called "Human Qi" (Ren Qi, 人氣).

Qi is also commonly used to express the energy state of something, especially living things. As mentioned before, the weather is called "Heaven Qi" (Tian Qi, 天氣) because it indicates the energy state of the heavens. When something is alive it has "Vital Qi" (Huo Qi, 活氣), and when it is dead it has "Dead Qi" (Si Qi, 死氣) or "Ghost Qi" (Gui Qi, 鬼氣). When a person is righteous and has the spiritual strength to do good, he is said to have "Normal Qi or Righteous Qi" (Zheng Qi, 正氣). The spiritual state or morale of an army is called "Energy state" (Qi Shi, 氣勢).

You can see that the word "Qi" has a wider and more general definition than most people think. It does not only refer to the energy circulating in the human body.

Furthermore, the word "Qi" can represent the energy itself, and it can even be used to express the manner or state of the energy. It is important to understand this when you practice Qigong, so that your mind is not channeled into a narrow understanding of Qi, which would limit your future understanding and development.

A Narrow Definition of Qi 氣的狹義

Now that you have read about the general definition of Qi, let us look at how Qi is defined in Qigong society today. As mentioned before, among the Three Powers, the Chinese have been most concerned with the Qi which is related to our health and longevity. Therefore, after four thousand years of emphasizing Human Qi, when people mention Qi they usually mean only the Qi circulating in our bodies.

If we look at Chinese medical and Qigong documents that were written about two thousand years ago, the word "Qi" was written " 炁 " This character is constructed of two words, " 旡 " on the top, which means "nothing;" and " 灬 " on the bottom, which means "fire". This means that the word "Qi" was actually written as "no fire" in ancient times. If we go back through Chinese medical and Qigong history, it is not hard to understand this expression.

In ancient times, the Chinese physicians or Qigong practitioners were actually looking for the Yin-Yang balance of the Qi which was circulating in the body. When this goal was reached, there was "no fire" in the internal organs. This concept is very simple. According to Chinese medicine, each of our internal organs needs to receive a specific amount of Qi to function properly. If an organ receives an improper amount of Qi (usually too much, i.e. too Yang), it will start to malfunction, and, in time, physical damage will occur. Therefore, the goal of the medical or Qigong practitioner was to attain a state of "no fire," which eventually became the word "Qi."

However, in more recent publications, the Qi of "no fire" has been replaced by the word " 氣 " which is again constructed of two words, " 气 " which means "air," and " 米 " which means "rice." This shows that later practitioners realized that the Qi circulating in our bodies is produced mainly by the breathing of air and the consumption of food (rice). Air is called "Kong Qi" (空氣), which literally means "space energy."

For a long time, people were confused about just what type of energy was circulating in our bodies. Many people believed that it was heat, others considered it to be electricity, and many others assumed that it was a mixture of heat, electricity, and light.

This confusion lasted until the early 1980's, when the concept of Qi gradually became clear. If we think carefully about what we know from science today, we can see that (except possibly for gravity) there is actually only one type of energy in this universe, and that is electromagnetic energy. This means that light (electromagnetic waves) and heat (infrared waves) are also part of electromagnetic energy. This makes it very clear that the Qi circulating in our bodies is actually "bioelectricity," and that our body is a "living electromagnetic field."[1] This field is affected by our thoughts, feelings, activities, the food we eat, the quality of the air we breathe, our lifestyle, the natural energy that surrounds us, and also the unnatural energy which modern life inflicts upon us.

Next, let us define Qigong. Once you understand what Qigong is, you will be able to better understand the role Qigong plays in Chinese medical science.

A General Definition of Qigong 氣功的廣義

We have explained that Qi is energy, and that it is found in the heavens, in the earth, and in every living thing. The word "Gong" (功) is often used instead of "Gongfu" (or Kung Fu, 功夫), which means energy and time. Any study or training which requires much energy and time to learn or to accomplish is called Gongfu. The term can be applied to any special skill or study as long as it requires time, energy, and patience. Therefore, the correct definition of Qigong is any training or study dealing with Qi which takes a long time and a lot of effort. You can see from this definition that Qigong is a scientific discipline which studies the energy in nature. The main difference between this energy science and Western energy science is that Qigong focuses on the inner energy of human beings, while Western energy science pays more attention to the energy outside of the human body. When you study Qigong, it is worthwhile to also consider the modern, scientific point of view, and not restrict yourself to only the traditional beliefs.

The Chinese have studied Qi for thousands of years. Some of the information on the patterns and cycles of nature has been recorded in books, one of which is the *Yi Jing* (易經) (*Book of Changes*; 1122 B.C.). When the *Yi Jing* was written, the Chinese people, as mentioned earlier, believed that natural power included Heaven (Tian, 天), Earth (Di, 地), and Man (Ren, 人). These are called the "Three Powers" (San Cai, 三才) and are manifested by the three Qi's: Heaven Qi, Earth Qi, and Human Qi. These three facets of nature have their definite rules and cycles. The rules never change, and the cycles repeat regularly. The Chinese people used an understanding of these natural principles and the *Yi Jing* to calculate the changes in natural Qi. This calculation is called the "Eight Trigrams" (Bagua, 八卦). From the Eight Trigrams are derived the 64 hexagrams. Therefore, the *Yi Jing* was probably the first book that taught the Chinese people about Qi and its variations in nature and man. The relationship of the three natural powers and their Qi variations were later discussed extensively in the book *Theory of Qi's Variation* (*Qi Hua Lun*, 氣化論).

Understanding Heaven Qi is very difficult, and it was especially so in ancient times when the science was just developing. But since nature is always repeating itself, the experiences accumulated over the years made it possible to trace the natural patterns. Understanding the rules and cycles of "heavenly timing" (Tian Shi, 天時) will help you to understand natural changes of the seasons, climate, weather, rain, snow, drought, and all other natural occurrences. If you observe carefully, you will be able to see many of these routine patterns and cycles caused by the rebalancing of the Qi fields. Among the natural cycles are those which repeat every day, month, or year, as well as cycles of twelve years and sixty years.

Earth Qi is a part of Heaven Qi. If you can understand the rules and the structure of the earth, you will be able to understand how mountains and rivers are formed, how plants grow, how rivers move, what part of the country is best for someone, where to build a house and which direction it should face so that it is a healthy place to live, and many other things related to the earth. In China today there are people, called "geomancy teachers" (Di Li Shi, 地理師) or "wind water teachers" (Feng Shui Shi, 風水師), who make their living this way. The term "wind water" (Feng Shui, 風水) is commonly used because the location and character of the wind and water in a landscape are the most important factors in evaluating a location. These experts use the accumulated body of geomantic knowledge and the Yi Jing (易經) to help people make important decisions such as where and how to build a house, where to bury their dead, and how to rearrange or redecorate homes and offices so that they are better places in which to live and work. Many people even believe that setting up a store or business according to the guidance of Feng Shui can make it more prosperous.

Among the three Qi's, Human Qi is probably the one studied most thoroughly. The study of Human Qi covers a large number of different subjects. The Chinese people believe that Human Qi is affected and controlled by Heaven Qi and Earth Qi, and that they in fact determine your destiny. Therefore, if you understand the relationship between nature and people, in addition to understanding "human relations" (Ren Shi, 人事), you will be able to predict wars, the destiny of a country, a person's desires and temperament, and even their future. The people who practice this profession are called calculate life teachers (Suan Ming Shi, 算命師).

However, the greatest achievement in the study of Human Qi is with regard to health and longevity. Since Qi is the source of life, if you understand how Qi functions and know how to regulate it correctly, you should be able to live a long and healthy life. Remember that you are part of nature, and you are channeled into the cycles of nature. If you go against this natural cycle, you may become sick, so it is in your best interest to follow the way of nature. This is the meaning of "Dao" (道) which can be translated as "The Natural Way."

Many different methods of Human Qi have been researched, using acupuncture, acupressure, massage, herbal treatment, meditation, and Qigong exercises. The use of acupuncture, acupressure, and herbal treatment to adjust Human Qi flow has become the foundation of Chinese medical science. Meditation and moving Qigong exercises are used widely by the Chinese people to improve their health or even to cure certain illnesses. In addition, Daoists and Buddhists use meditation and Qigong exercises in their pursuit of enlightenment and Buddhahood.

In conclusion, the study of any of the aspects of Qi including Heaven Qi, Earth Qi, and Human Qi should be called Qigong. However, since the term is usually used today only in reference to the cultivation of Human Qi through meditation and exercises, we will only use it in this narrower sense to avoid confusion.

A Narrow Definition of Qigong 氣功的狹義

As mentioned earlier, the narrow definition of Qi is "the energy circulating in the human body." Therefore, the narrow definition of Qigong is "the study of the Qi circulating in the human body." Because our bodies are part of nature, the narrow definition of Qigong should also include the study of how our bodies relate to Heaven Qi and Earth Qi. Chinese Qigong consists today of several different fields: acupuncture, herbs for regulating Human Qi, martial arts Qigong, Qigong massage, Qigong exercises, Qigong healing, and religious enlightenment Qigong. Naturally, these fields are mutually related, and in many cases cannot be separated.

The Chinese have discovered that the human body has twelve major Qi Channels (Shi Er Jing, 十二經) and Eight Vessels (Ba Mai, 八脈) through which the Qi circulates. The twelve channels are like *rivers* which distribute Qi throughout the body, and also connect the extremities (fingers and toes) to the internal organs. Here you should understand that the "internal organs" of Chinese medicine do not necessarily correspond to the physical organs as understood in the West, but rather to a set of clinical functions similar to each other and related to the organ system. The eight vessels, which are often referred to as the extraordinary vessels, function like reservoirs and regulate the distribution and circulation of Qi in your body.

When the Qi in the eight reservoirs is full and strong, the Qi in the rivers is strong and is regulated efficiently. When there is stagnation in any of these twelve channels or rivers, the Qi which flows to the body's extremities and to the internal organs is abnormal, and illness may develop. You should understand that every channel has its particular Qi flow strength, and every channel is different. All of these different levels of Qi strength are affected by your mind, the weather, the time of day, the food you have eaten, and even your mood. For example, when the weather is dry, the Qi in the lungs will tend to be more positive than when it is moist. When you are angry, the Qi flow in your Liver Channel will be abnormal. The Qi strength in the different channels varies throughout the day in a regular cycle, and at any particular time one channel is strongest. For example, between 11 A.M. and 1 P.M. the Qi flow in the Heart Channel is the strongest. Furthermore, the Qi level in the same organ can be different from one person to another.[2]

Whenever the Qi flow in the twelve rivers or channels is not normal, the eight reservoirs regulates the Qi flow and returns it to normal. For example, when you experience a sudden shock, the Qi flow in the bladder immediately becomes deficient. Normally, the reservoir immediately regulates the Qi in this channel so that you recover from the shock. However, if the reservoir Qi is also deficient, or if the effect of the shock is too great and there is not enough time to regulate the Qi, the bladder suddenly contracts, causing unavoidable urination.

When a person is sick, his Qi level tends to be either too positive (excessive) (Yang, 陽) or too negative (deficient) (Yin, 陰). A Chinese physician would either use a prescription of herbs to adjust the Qi, or else he would insert acupuncture needles at various spots on the channels to inhibit the flow in some channels and stimulate the flow in others, so that balance could be restored. However, there is another alternative, and that is to use certain physical and mental exercises to adjust the Qi. In other words, to use Qigong.

The above discussion is only to offer an idea of the narrow definition of Qigong. In fact, when people talk about Qigong today, most of the time they are referring to the mental and physical exercises that work with Qi.

A Modern Definition of Qi 氣的現代定義

It is important that you know about the progress that has been made by modern science in the study of Qi. This will keep you from getting stuck in the ancient concepts and level of understanding.

In ancient China, people had very little knowledge of electricity. They only knew from acupuncture that when a needle was inserted into an acupuncture cavity, some kind of energy other than heat was produced that often caused a shock or a tickling sensation. It was not until the last few decades, when the Chinese people were more acquainted with electromagnetic science, that they began to recognize that this energy circulating in the body, which they called Qi, might be the same thing as what today's science calls "bioelectricity".

It is understood now that the human body is constructed of many different electrically conductive materials, and that it forms a living electromagnetic field and circuit. Electromagnetic energy is continuously being generated in the human body through the biochemical reaction in food and air assimilation, and circulated by the electromotive forces (EMF) generated within the body.

In addition, you are constantly being affected by external electromagnetic fields such as that of the earth or the electrical fields generated by clouds. When you practice Chinese medicine or Qigong, you need to be aware of these outside factors and take them into account.

Countless experiments have been conducted in China, Japan, and other countries to study how external magnetic or electrical fields can affect and adjust the body's Qi field. Many acupuncturists use magnets and electricity in their treatments. They attach a magnet to the skin over a cavity and leave it there for a period of time. The magnetic field gradually affects the Qi circulation in that channel. Alternatively, they insert needles into cavities, and then run an electric current through the needle to reach the Qi channels directly. Although many researchers have claimed a degree of success in their experiments, none has been able to publish any detailed and convincing proof of the results, or give a good explanation of the theory behind the experiment. As with many other attempts to explain the *How* and *Why* of acupuncture, conclusive proof is elusive, and many unanswered questions remain. Of course, this theory is quite new, and it will probably take much more study and research before it is verified and completely understood. At present, there are many conservative acupuncturists who remain skeptical.

To untie this knot, we must look at what modern Western science has discovered about bioelectromagnetic energy. Many related bioelectricity reports have been published, and frequently the results are closely related to what is experienced in Chinese Qigong training and medical science. For example, when electrophysiological research was done during the 1960's, several investigators discovered that bones are piezoelectric; that is, when they are stressed, mechanical energy is converted to electrical energy in the form of electric current.[1] This might explain one of the practices of Marrow Washing Qigong in which the stress on the bones and muscles is increased in certain ways to increase the Qi circulation.

Dr. Robert O. Becker has done important work in this field. His book *The Body Electric* reports on much of the research concerning the body's electric field.[2] It is presently believed that food and air are the fuels which generate the electricity in the body through biochemical reactions. This electricity, that is circulated throughout the entire body by means of electrically conductive tissue, is one of the main energy sources that keep the cells of the physical body alive.

Whenever you have an injury or are sick, your body's electrical circulation is affected. If this circulation of electricity stops, you die. But bioelectric energy not only maintains life, it is also responsible for repairing physical damage. Many researchers have sought ways to use external electrical or magnetic fields to speed up the body's recovery from physical injury. Richard Leviton reports "Researchers at Loma Linda University's School of medicine in California have found, following studies in sixteen countries with over 1,000 patients, that low-frequency, low-intensity magnetic energy has been successful in treating chronic pain related to tissue ischemia, and has also worked in clearing up slow-healing ulcers, and in 90 percent of patients tested, raised blood flow significantly."[3]

Mr. Leviton also reports that every cell of the body functions like an electric battery and is able to store electric charges. He adds that "Other biomagnetic investigators take an even closer look to find out what is happening, right down to the level of the blood, the organs, and the individual cell, which they regard as 'a small electric battery'."[3] This has convinced me that our entire body is essentially a large battery which is assembled from millions of small batteries. All of these batteries together form the human electromagnetic field.

Furthermore, much of the research on the body's electrical field relates to acupuncture. For example, Dr. Becker reports that the conductivity of the skin is much higher at acupuncture cavities, and that it is now possible to locate them precisely by measuring the skin's conductivity (Figure 1-1).[2] Many of these reports prove that the acupuncture which has been done in China for thousands of years has a reasonable and scientific basis.

Some researchers use the theory of the body's electricity to explain many of the ancient "miracles" that have been attributed to the practice of Qigong. A report by Albert L. Huebner states that "These demonstrations of body electricity in human

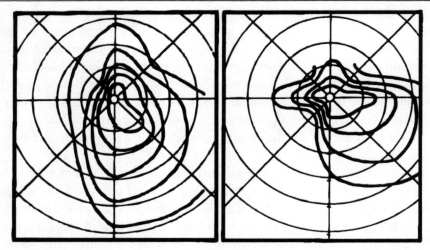

FIGURE 1-1. ELECTRICAL CONDUCTIVITY MAPS OF THE SKIN SURFACE OVER ACUPUNCTURE POINTS

beings may also offer a new explanation of an ancient healing practice. If weak external fields can produce powerful physiological effects, it may be that fields from human tissues in one person are capable of producing clinical improvements in another. In short, the method of healing known as the laying on of hands could be an especially subtle form of electrical stimulation."[1]

Another frequently reported phenomenon is that when a Qigong practitioner has reached a high level of development, a corona or halo would appear behind and/or around his head during meditation. This is commonly seen in paintings of Jesus Christ, the Buddha, and various Oriental immortals. Frequently the light is pictured as surrounding the whole body. This phenomenon may again be explained by the Body Electric theory. When a person has cultivated their Qi (electricity) to a high level, the Qi may be led to accumulate in the head. This Qi may then interact with the oxygen molecules in the air, and ionize them, causing them to glow.

Although the link between the theory of *The Body Electric* and the Chinese theory of Qi is becoming more accepted and better proven, there are still many questions to be answered. For example, how can the mind lead Qi (electricity)? How does the mind actually generate an EMF (electromotive force) to circulate the electricity in the body? How is the human electromagnetic field affected by the multitude of other electric fields that surround us, such as radio wiring or electrical appliances? How can we readjust our electromagnetic fields and survive in outer space or on other planets where the magnetic field is completely different from the earth's? You can see that the future of Qigong and bioelectric science is a challenging and exciting one. It is about time that we started to use modern technology to understand the inner energy world which has been for the most part ignored by Western society.

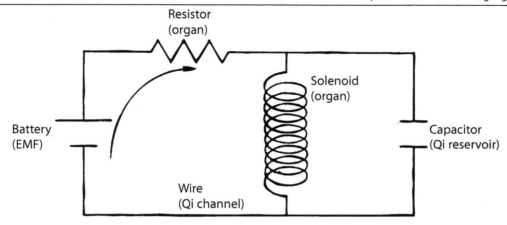

FIGURE 1-2. THE HUMAN BIOELECTRIC CIRCUIT IS SIMILAR TO AN ELECTRIC CIRCUIT

A Modern Definition of Qigong 氣功的現代定義

If you now accept that the inner energy (Qi) circulating in our bodies is bioelectricity, then we can now formulate a definition of Qigong based on principles of electricity.

Let us assume that the circuit shown in Figure 1-2 is similar to the circuit in our bodies. Unfortunately, although we now have a certain degree of understanding of this circuit from acupuncture, we still do not know in detail exactly what the body's circuit looks like. We know that there are twelve primary Qi Channels (Qi rivers) (Jing, 經) and Eight Vessels (Qi reservoirs) (Mai, 脈) in our body. There are also thousands of small secondary Qi channels (streams) (Luo, 絡) that branch out from the primary channels to reach the skin surface and the bone marrow. Consequently, the Qi can be transported to the skin surface (Guardian Qi) (Wei Qi, 衛氣) and also to the bone marrow (Marrow Qi) (Sui Qi, 髓氣). In this circuit, the twelve internal organs are connected and mutually related through these secondary channels.

If you look at the electrical circuit in the illustration, you will see that:

1. The Qi channels are like the wires that carry electric current.
2. The internal organs are like the electrical components such as resistors and solenoids.
3. The Qi vessels are like capacitors (i.e., regulators), that regulate the current in the circuit.
4. The Lower Dan Tian (Xia Dan Tian, 下丹田) is like the battery that produces and stores the Qi.

How do you keep this electrical circuit functioning most efficiently? Your first concern is the resistance of the wire which carries the current. In a machine, you want to use a wire which has a high level of conductivity and low resistance, otherwise the current may melt the wire. Therefore, the wire should be of a material like copper or perhaps even gold. In your body, you want to keep the current flowing smoothly. This means that your first task is to remove anything which interferes with the flow and causes stagnation. Fat has low conductivity, so you should use diet and exercise to remove excess fat from your body. You should also learn how to relax your physical body, because this opens all of the Qi channels. This is why relaxation is the first goal in Taijiquan and many Qigong exercises.

Your next concern in maintaining a healthy electrical circuit is the amount of current going through the components—your internal organs. If you do not have the correct level of current in your organs, they will either burn out from too much current (Yang, 陽) or malfunction because of a deficient level of current (Yin, 陰). In order to avoid these problems in a machine, you would use a capacitor to regulate the current. Whenever there is too much current, the capacitor absorbs and stores the excess, and whenever the current is weak, the capacitor supplies current to raise the level. The Eight Qi Vessels are your body's capacitors. Qigong is concerned with learning how to increase the level of Qi in these vessels so that they will be able to supply current when needed, and keep the internal organs functioning smoothly. This is especially important as you get older and your Qi level is generally lower.

Finally, in order to maintain a healthy circuit, you have to be concerned with the components themselves. If any of them are not strong and of good quality, the entire circuit will have problems. This means that the final concern in Qigong practice is maintaining or even rebuilding the health of your internal organs. Before we go any further, we should point out that there is an important difference between the circuit shown in the diagram and the Qi circuit in our bodies. This difference is that the human body is alive, and with the proper Qi nourishment, all of the cells can be regrown and the state of health improved. For example, if you can jog about three miles today, and if you keep jogging regularly and gradually increase the distance, eventually you will be able to jog five miles easily. This is because your body rebuilds and readjusts itself to fit the circumstances.

If we can increase the Qi flow through our internal organs, they can become stronger and healthier. Naturally, the increase in Qi must be slow and gradual so that the organs can adjust to it. In order to increase the Qi flow in your body, you need to work with the EMF (electromotive force) in your body. If you do not know what EMF is, imagine two containers filled with water and connected by a tube. If both containers have the same water level, then the water will not flow. However, if one side is higher than the other, the water will flow from that container to the other. In electricity, this potential difference is called electromotive force. Naturally, the higher the EMF is, the stronger the current will flow.

You can see from this discussion that the key to effective Qigong practice is, in addition to removing resistance from the Qi channels and increasing Qi quantity, learning how to increase the EMF in your body. Now let us see what the sources of EMF in the body are, so that we may use them to increase the flow of bioelectricity. Generally speaking, there are five major sources:

1. Natural Energy. Since your body is constructed of electrically conductive material, its electromagnetic field is always affected by the sun, the moon, clouds, the earth's magnetic field, and by the other energies around you. The major influences are the sun's radiation, the moon's gravity, and the earth's magnetic field. These affect your Qi circulation significantly and are responsible for the pattern of your Qi circulation since you were formed. We are now also being greatly affected by the energy generated by modern technology, such as the electromagnetic waves generated by radio, TV, microwave ovens, computers, and many other things. If you would like to know more about this energy pollution, please refer to the book: *Cross Currents*, by Dr. Robert O. Becker.

2. Food and Air. In order to maintain life, we take in food and air essence through our mouth and nose. These essences are then converted into Qi through biochemical reaction in the chest and digestive system (called the Triple Burner in Chinese medicine). When Qi is converted from the essence, an EMF is generated that circulates the Qi throughout the body. Consequently a major part of Qigong is devoted to obtaining the proper kinds of food and fresh air. Through years of study, the Chinese have discovered many kinds of herbs, such as Ginseng (Ren Shen, 人參), that are able to increase the quantity of the Qi and enhance the Qi circulation in the body.

3. Thinking. The human mind is the most important and efficient source of bio-electric EMF. Any time you move to do something, you must first generate an idea (Yi, 意). This idea generates the EMF and leads the Qi to energize the appropriate muscles to carry out the desired motion. The more you can concentrate, the stronger the EMF you can generate, and the stronger the flow of Qi you can lead. Naturally, the stronger the flow of Qi you lead to the muscles, the more they will be energized. Because of this, the mind is considered the most important factor in Qigong training.

4. Exercise. Exercise converts the food essence (fat) stored in your body into Qi, and therefore builds up the EMF. Many Qigong styles have been created which utilize movement for this purpose. Furthermore, when you exercise, you are also using your mind to manage your physical body, and this enhances the EMF for the Qi's circulation.

5. Converting Pre-Birth Essence into Qi. The hormones produced by our endocrine glands are referred to as "Pre-Birth Essence" in Chinese medicine.

These hormones regulate the body's metabolic processes. This also means helping the body's biochemical reactions be carried out smoothly. When this happens, the food eaten or the fat stored in the body can be converted into Qi more efficiently, thus stimulating the functioning of our physical body and increasing vitality. Balancing hormone production when you are young and increasing its production when you are old are important concerns in Chinese Qigong.

6. Artificial Methods. Chinese medical and Qigong practices teaches us that through acupuncture, acupressure, massage, and artificial electromagnetic stimulation, the body's Qi can be regulated into a balanced state. This is the root of Chinese healing medical care. However, as mentioned earlier, we cannot deny that since the 1940's much artificial radiation (i.e. energy pollution) has been created and has influenced the Qi's circulation in our bodies. This energy pollution is a risk to health, and has caused many serious illnesses, such as cancer. Again, if you wish to know more about energy pollution, please refer to the book: *Cross Currents*, by Dr. Robert O. Becker.

The key to increasing the Qi quantity is to generate more Qi at the Lower Dan Tian (biobattery) and store higher levels of it. The first step to reaching this goal is to condition the biobattery. If your battery is the same as others, how can you expect the storage of your Qi to be greater than others? Through more than fifteen hundred years of study and practice, the Chinese have realized that conditioning this battery is best accomplished through Muscle/Tendon Changing and Marrow/Brain Washing Qigong. To generate and store more Qi at the biobattery, you must know the methods of abdominal breathing and embryonic breathing. If you wish to know more about these subjects, please refer to the books: *Qigong—The Secret of Youth* and also *Qigong Meditation—Embryonic Breathing*.

From the foregoing, you can see that within the human body, there is a network of electrical circuitry. You can achieve health and longevity by increasing the Qi's storage so the Qi's circulation is enhanced. In order to reach this goal, you must know about the biobattery in your body. Where then, is the biobattery?

Chinese Qigong practitioners believe that there is a place which is able to store Qi (bioelectricity). This place is called the Dan Tian (i.e., elixir field). According to such practitioners, there are three Dan Tians in the human body. One is located at the abdominal area, one or two inches below the navel and is called the "Lower Dan Tian" (Xia Dan Tian, 下丹田). The second is in the area of the lower sternum and is called the "Middle Dan Tian" (Zhong Dan Tian, 中丹田). The third is the lower center of forehead (or the third eye), connected to the brain and is called the "Upper Dan Tian" (Shang Dan Tian, 上丹田).

The Lower Dan Tian is considered to be the residence of the Water Qi, or the Qi

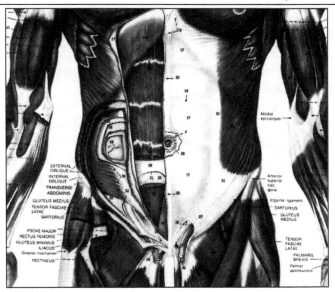

FIGURE 1-3. ANATOMIC STRUCTURE OF THE ABDOMINAL AREA

that is generated from the Original Essence (Yuan Jing, 元精). Therefore, Qi stored here is called Original Qi (Yuan Qi, 元氣). According to Chinese medicine, in this same area there is a cavity called "Qihai" (Co-6) (氣海), which means "Qi ocean." This is consistent with the conclusions drawn by Qigong practitioners, who also call this area the "Lower Dan Tian" (lower elixir field). Both groups agree that this area is able to produce Qi or elixir like a field, and that here the Qi is abundant like an ocean.

In Qigong practice, it is well known that in order to build up the Qi to a higher level in the Lower Dan Tian, you must move your abdominal area (i.e. Lower Dan Tian) up and down through abdominal breathing. This kind of up and down abdominal breathing exercise is called "Qi Huo" (起火) and means "start the fire." It is also called "back to childhood breathing" (Fan Tong Hu Xi, 返童呼吸). Normally, after you have exercised the Lower Dan Tian for about ten minutes, you will have a feeling of warmth in the lower abdomen, which implies the accumulation of Qi or energy.

Theoretically and scientifically, what is happening when the abdominal area is moved up and down? If you look at the structure of the abdominal area, you will see that there are about six layers of muscle and fasciae sandwiching each other in this area (Figure 1-3). In fact, what you actually see is the sandwich of muscles and fat accumulated in the fasciae layers. When you move your abdomen up and down, you are actually using your mind to move the muscles, not the fat. Whenever there is a muscular contraction and relaxation, the fat slowly turns into bioelectricity. When this bioelectricity encounters resistance from the fasciae layers, it turns into heat. From this, you can see how simple the theory might be for the generation of Qi. Another thing you should know is that, according to our understanding today, fat and fasciae are poor electrical conductors, while the muscles are relatively good electrical conductors.[1,2,3] When these good and poor electrical materials are sandwiched together, they act like a battery. This is why, through up and down abdominal movements, the energy can be stored temporarily and generate warmth.

However, through nearly two thousand years of experience, Daoists have said that the front abdominal area is not the Real Dan Tian, but is in fact a "False Dan Tian" (Jia Dan Tian, 假丹田). Their argument is that, although this Lower Dan Tian is able to generate Qi and build it up to a higher level, it does not store it for a long time. This is because the Lower Dan Tian is located on the path of the Conception Vessel (please refer to the next chapter about vessels), so that whenever Qi is built up to a higher energetic state, it will circulate in the Conception and Governing Vessels. According to Chinese medicine, these two vessels regulate and govern the Qi conditions in the body's twelve primary Qi channels. Therefore, when there is any extra Qi in these two vessels, the Qi will eventually redistribute to the entire body through the twelve channels. This Lower Dan Tian therefore cannot be a battery as we understand the term. A real battery should be able to store the Qi to an abundant level. Where then is the "Real Dan Tian" (Zhen Dan Tian, 真丹田)?

Daoists teach that the Real Dan Tian is at the center of the abdominal area, at the physical center of the gravity located in the large and small intestines (Figure 1-4). Now, let us analyze this from two different points of view.

First, let us take a look of how a life is started. It begins with a sperm from the father entering an egg from the mother, thus forming the original human cell (Figure 1-5).[4] This cell next divides into two cells, then four cells, and so forth. When this group of cells adheres to the internal wall of the uterus, the umbilical cord starts to develop. Nutrition and energy for further cell multiplication is absorbed through the umbilical cord from the mother's body. The baby keeps growing until matured. During this period of nourishment and growth, the baby's abdomen is moving up and down, acting like a pump drawing in nutrition and energy into his or her body. Later, immediately after the birth, air and nutrition are taken in from the nose and mouth through the mouth's sucking action and the lungs' breathing. As the child grows, it slowly forgets the natural movements of the abdomen. This is why the abdomen's up and down movement is called "back to childhood breathing" (Fan Tong Hu Xi, 返童呼吸)

Think carefully: If your first human cell is still alive, where is this cell? Naturally, this cell has already died a long time ago. It is understood that approximately one trillion (10^{12}) cells die in a human body each day.[5] However, if we assume that this first cell is still alive, then it should be located at our physical center, that is, our center of gravity. If we think carefully, we can see that it is from this center that the cells could multiply evenly outward until the body is completely constructed. In order to maintain this even multiplication physically, the energy or Qi must be centered at this point and radiate

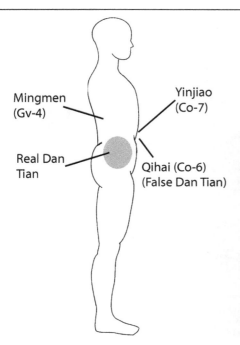

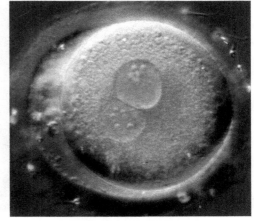

FIGURE 1-4. THE REAL DAN TIAN
AND THE FALSE DAN TIAN

FIGURE 1-5. ORIGINAL FIRST HUMAN CELL

outward. When we are in an embryonic state, this is the gravity center and also the Qi center. As we grow after birth, this center remains.

The above argument adheres solely to the traditional point of view of the physical development of our body. Next, let us analyze this center from another point of view.

If we look at the physical center of gravity, we can see that the entire area is occupied by the large and small intestines (Figure 1-6). We know that there are three kinds of muscles existing in our body and can examine them in ascending order of our ability to control them. The first kind is the heart muscle, in which the electrical conductivity among muscular groups is the highest. The heart beats all the time, regardless of our attention. Through practice and discipline, we are able only to regulate its beating, not start and stop it. If we supply electricity to even a small piece of this muscle, it will pump like the heart. The second category of muscles are those which contract automatically but slowly, such as the muscles in the large and small intestines, and their electrical conductivity is lower than the first type. The third kind of muscles are those muscles that are directly controlled by our conscious mind. The electric conductivity of these muscles is the lowest of the three groups.

If you look at the structure of the large and small Intestines, the first thing you notice is that the total length of your large and small Intestines is approximately six times your body's height (Figure 1-7). With such long electrically conductive tissues sand-

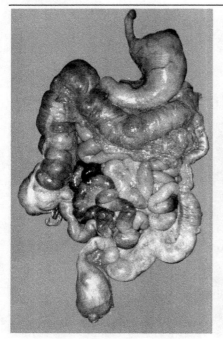

FIGURE 1-6. ANATOMIC STRUCTURE
OF THE REAL DAN TIAN

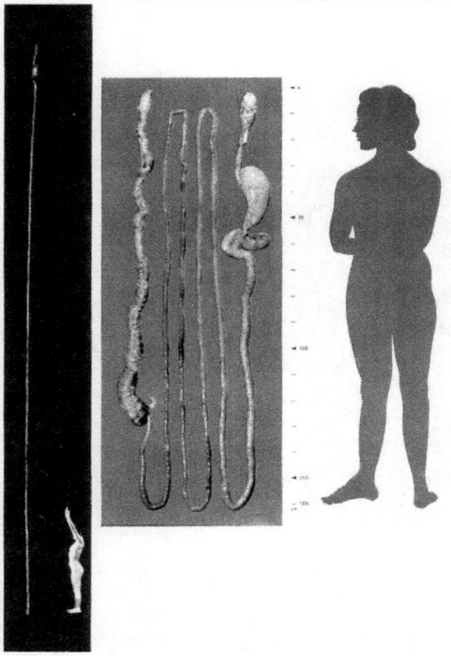

FIGURE 1-7. THE LARGE AND SMALL INTESTINES
ARE ABOUT SIX TIMES YOUR HEIGHT

wiched between all of the mesentery, water, and outer casings (which it is reasonable to believe are poor electrical conductive tissues), these organs act like a huge battery in our body (Figure 1-8).[6] From this, you can see that it makes sense both logically and scientifically that the center of gravity, rather than the False Dan Tian, is the real battery in our body.

Next, let us examine the structure of the Middle Dan Tian area. The Middle Dan Tian is located next to the diaphragm (Figure 1-9). We know that the diaphragm is a membranous muscular partition separating the abdominal and the thoracic cavities. It functions in respiration and is a good electrically conductive material. On the top and the bottom of the diaphragm there are the fasciae, which isolates the internal organs from the diaphragm. We see now again a good electrical conductor isolated by a poor electrical conductor. That means that the fasciae are capable of storing electricity or Qi. Since they are between the lungs and the stomach, and they absorb the Post-Birth essence (air and food) and convert it into energy, the Qi accumulated in the Middle Dan Tian is classified as Fire Qi (Huo Qi, 火氣). The reason for this name is that the Qi converted from the contaminated air and the food can affect Qi status and make it Yang. Naturally, this Fire Qi can also agitate your emotional mind.

Finally, let us analyze the brain, which is considered the Upper Dan Tian. We already know that the brain and the spinal cord are considered to be the central nervous

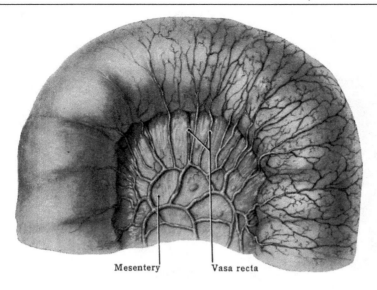

FIGURE 1-8. LOW ELECTRICALLY CONDUCTIVE MATERIALS SUCH AS MESENTERY, OUTER CASING, AND WATER IN AND AROUND THE INTESTINES MAKES THE ENTIRE AREA ACT LIKE A BATTERY
(James E. Anderson, M.D., *Grant's Atlas of Anatomy*, 7th ed., © Williams & Wilkins)

system, in which the electrical conductivity is highest in our body. If we examine the brain's structure, we can see that it is segregated by the arachnoid mater (i.e. a delicate membrane of the spinal cord and brain, lying between the pia mater and dura mater) into separate portions (Figure 1-10). It is reasonable to assume that these materials are low electrically conductive tissues. Again, the brain is another giant battery which consumes Qi in great amounts. However, since the brain does not produce Qi or bioelectricity, its function as a Dan Tian cannot be considered to be the same as the Lower Dan Tian.

From the above discussion, you may have gained a better idea of how we can link ancient experience together with modern scientific understanding. Recently, scientists have even discovered that we have two "brains" coexisting in

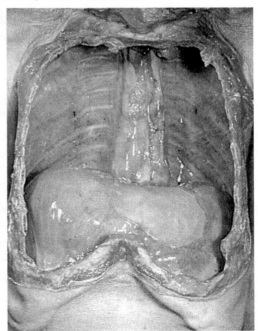

FIGURE 1-9. THE MIDDLE DAN TIAN IS CONNECTED TO THE DIAPHRAGM

our body. One is the head, as we have known for quite some time. The other is actual-

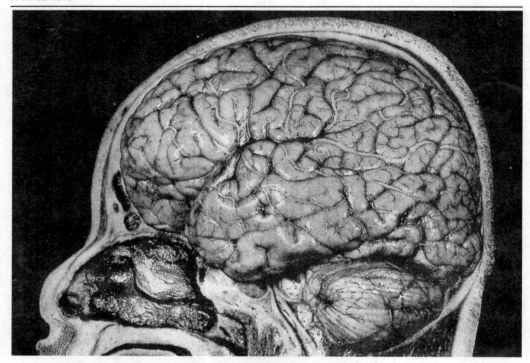

FIGURE 1-10. THE UPPER DAN TIAN—THE HUMAN BRAIN

ly in the gut. These scientists have confirmed that the upper brain is able to think and store memory. However, the lower brain is believed capable of storing memory only. These two brains are connected and communicate with each other through the spinal cord (i.e. Thrusting Vessel; Chong Mai, 衝脈), a very highly electrically conductive nerve fiber. Therefore, while physically there are two brains, in function, they act as one unit. The upper brain thinks and generates EMF, and the lower brain stores charges and supplies electricity through the spinal cord.[7]

This is very consistent with the Chinese discoveries discussed earlier. As mentioned previously, according to Chinese Qigong, the upper brain is our Upper Dan Tian, where the spirit resides and the mind functions, while the Lower Dan Tian in the gut (i.e. stomach, large and small intestines) is the place that stores and supplies Qi. From this, you can clearly see that both Chinese empirical experience and modern science agree that the more you can concentrate, the higher your EMF will be. This will lead to more electricity being led from the Lower Dan Tian through the spinal cord (i.e. Thrusting Vessel) to anywhere in your physical body for action.

In order to make the scientific concept of Qigong even more clear, let us look at Qigong from another scientific point of view, this time chemical.

If we examine how we breath, we can see that we inhale to take in oxygen, and we exhale to expel carbon dioxide (Figure 1-11). From this, we can see that every minute

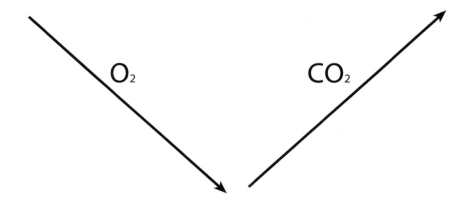

O_2 CO_2

FIGURE 1-11. WE INHALE TO ABSORB OXYGEN AND EXHALE TO EXPEL CARBON DIOXIDE

we expel a great deal of carbon from our body through exhalation. Carbon is a material in a physical form that can be seen. The question is, where is the carbon coming from in our body? Through breathing, how much carbon is actually processed out?

The first source of carbon is from the food (glucose) we eat. When this food is converted into energy through chemical reaction during our daily activities, carbon dioxide is produced.[8]

$$\text{glucose} + 6O_2 \longrightarrow 6CO_2 + 6H_2O$$

$$\Delta G^{o'} = -686 \text{ Kcal}$$

Remember the Chinese word for Qi (氣) is constructed from two words: air (气) and rice (米). Air means oxygen, while rice is glucose. Air (Kong Qi, 空氣) is classified as Upper Level Qi (Shang Ceng Qi, 上層氣) since it is taken in by the lungs, which is above the diaphragm. This form of bioelectricity is considered to be Lower Level Qi (Xia Ceng Qi, 下層氣) because it is stored at the guts underneath the diaphragm. When 686 Kcal of energy is converted or transformed (i.e. manifested) in the body, it can manifest as heat, light, or bioelectricity. Heat and light do not circulate in the body, however, bioelectricity does. From this, we can see how the Qi is converted from food and air. This implies that what we eat and how we breathe are the crucial keys to Qigong practice.

The second source of this carbon is from dead cells in our body. We already know that the majority of our body is constructed from the elements Carbon (C), Hydrogen (H_2), Oxygen (O_2), and Nitrogen (N_2), while other elements such as Calcium (Ca), Phosphorus (P), Chloride (Cl), Sulfur (S), Potassium (K), Sodium (Na), Magnesium (Mg), Iodine (I), and Iron (Fe) comprise much less of our body weight. This means that the cells in our body contain a great amount of carbon.

In addition, consider that every cell in our body has a lifetime. As many as a trillion (10^{12}) cells die in our body every 24 hours.[5] For example, we know that the life span of a skin cell is 28 days. Naturally, every living cell such as those of the bone, marrow, liver, have their own individual lifetime. We rely on our respiration to bring the carbon (i.e. dead cells) out, and to supply living cells with new oxygen through inhalation, and new carbon sources, water, and other minerals from eating. All this aids in the formation of new cells and the continuation of life.

From the foregoing, we can conclude that the cell replacement process is ongoing at all times in our life. Health during our lifetime depends on how smoothly and how quickly this replacement process is carried out. If there are more new healthy cells to replace the old cells, you live and grow. If the cells replaced are as healthy as the original cells, you remain young. However, if there are fewer cells produced, or if the new cells are not as healthy as the original cells, then you age. Now, let us analyze Qigong from the point of view of cell replacement.

In order to produce a good, healthy cell, first you must consider the materials that are needed. From an understanding of the structure of a cell, we know that we will need hydrogen, oxygen, carbon, and other minerals which we can absorb either from air or food. Therefore, air quality, water purity, and the choice of foods become critical factors for your health and longevity. Naturally, this has also been a large component of Qigong study.

However, we know that air and water quality today has been contaminated by pollution. This is especially bad in big cities and industrial areas. The quality of the food we eat depends on their source and processing methods. Naturally, it is not easy to find the same pristine environments as in ancient times. However, we must learn how to fit into our new environment and choose the way of our life wisely.

Since carbon comprises such a major part of our body, how to absorb good quality carbon is an important issue in modern health. You may obtain carbon from animal products or from plants. Generally speaking, the carbon originating from plants is purer and cleaner than that taken from animals.

According to past experience and analysis, red meat is generally more contaminated than white meat, and is able to disturb and stimulate your emotional mind and confuse your thinking. Another source from which animal products can be obtained is fish. Again, some fish are good and others may be bad. For example, shrimp is high in cholesterol, which may increase your risk of high blood pressure.

In attempting to avoid the impurities contained in most animal products, Qigong practitioners since ancient times learned how to absorb protein from plants, especially from peas or beans. Soybean is one of the best of these sources; it is both inexpensive and easy to grow. However, if you are not a vegetarian originally, then it can be difficult for your body to produce the enzymes to digest an all-vegetable diet immediately. Humans evolved as omnivores, and the craving for meat can be strong. Even today, we all still have canine teeth, that are designed for the simple purpose of tearing flesh from bone. Therefore, the natural enzymes existing in our body are more tailored to digesting meat. In an experiment, if we place a piece of meat and some corn in human digestive enzymes, we will see that the meat will be dissolved in a matter of minutes, while the corn will take many hours. This means it is generally easier for a human to absorb meat rather than plants as a protein source.

However, the above discussion does not mean we cannot absolutely absorb plant protein efficiently. The key is that if it is present to begin with, the enzyme production can be increased within your body, but it will take time. For example, if you cannot drink milk due to insufficient lactaste enzyme in your stomach, you may start by drinking a little bit of milk every day, and slowly increase it as days pass by. You will realize that you can absorb milk six months later. This means that if you wish to become a vegetarian, you must reduce the intake of meat products slowly and allow your body to adjust to it; otherwise you may experience protein deficiency.

Other than a protein source, you must also consider minerals. Although they do not comprise a large proportion of our body, their importance in some ways is more significant than carbon. We know that calcium is an important element for bones, and iron is crucial for blood cells, etc. Therefore, when we eat we must consume a variety of foods instead of just a few. How to absorb nutrition from food has been an important part of Chinese Qigong study.

In order to produce healthy cells, other than the concerns of the material side, you must also consider energy. You should understand that when a person ages quickly, often it is not because he or she is malnourished, but instead results from the weakening of their Qi storage and circulation. Without an abundant supply of Qi (bioelectricity), Qi circulation will not be regulated efficiently, and therefore your life force will weaken and the physical body will degenerate. In order to attain abundant Qi storage, you must learn Qigong in order to build up the Qi in your eight vessels, and also to help you understand how to lead the Qi circulating in your body. This kind of Qigong training includes Wai Dan (外丹) (external elixir) and Nei Dan (內丹) (internal elixir) practice, which we will discuss in the next section.

Other than the concern for materials needed, and the Qi required for cell production and replacement, the next thing you should ask yourself is how this replacement process is carried out. Then, you will see that the entire replacement process depends on the blood cells. From Western medicine, we know that a blood cell is the carrier of water, oxygen, and nutrients to everywhere in the body through the blood circulatory network. From arteries and capillaries, the components for new cells are brought to every tiny place in the body. The old cells then absorb everything required from the blood stream and divide to produce new cells. The dead cells are brought back through veins where respiration occurs to the lungs. Through respiration, the dead cell materials are expelled from the body as carbon dioxide.

However, there is one thing missing from the last process. This is the Qi or bioelectricity which is required for the biochemical process of cell division. It has been proven that every blood cell is actually like a dipole or a small battery, which is able to store bioelectricity and also to release it.[1] This means that each blood cell is actually a carrier of Qi. This is also understood in Chinese medicine. In Chinese medicine, the blood and the Qi are always together. Where there is blood, there is Qi, and where there is Qi, the blood will also be there. Therefore, the term "Qi-Xue" (i.e. Qi blood) (氣血) is often used in Chinese medicine.

If you understand the above discussion, and if we take a look at our blood circulatory system, we can see that the arteries are located deeply underneath the muscles, while the veins are situated near the skin's surface. The color of the blood is red in the arteries because of the presence of oxygen, and its color is blue in the veins both because of the absence of this oxygen and the presence of carbon dioxide. This implies that cell replacement actually happens from inside of the body, moving outward. This can also offer us a hint that, if we tense more, the blood circulation will be more stagnant and cell replacement will be slower. We can also conclude that most cell replacement occurs in the night when we are at our most relaxed state, during sleep. This can further lead one to conclude the importance of sleeping.

If we already know that blood cells are the carriers of everything that is required for cell replacement, then we must also consider the health of our blood cells. If you have good health and a sufficient quantity of blood cells, then the nutrition and Qi can be carried to every part of the body efficiently. You will be healthy. However, if you do not have sufficient blood cells, or if the quality of the cells is poor, then the entire cell replacement process will be stagnant. Naturally, you will degenerate swiftly.

According to modern medical science, blood cells also have a life span. When the old ones die, new ones must be produced from the bone marrow. Bone marrow is the major blood factory. From medical reports, we know that normally, after a person reaches thirty, the marrow near the ends of the bone cavity turns yellow. This indicates that fat has accumulated there. It also means that red blood cells are no longer being produced in the yellowed area (Figure 1-12).[9] Chinese Qigong practitioners believe that the degeneration of the bone marrow is due to insufficient Qi supply. Therefore, Bone Marrow Washing Qigong was developed. From experience, through Marrow Washing Qigong practice, health can be improved and life can be extended significantly. If you are interested in this subject, please read *Qigong—Secret of Youth*, by Dr. Yang, Jwing-Ming.

In addition to the above, the next thing which is highly important in human life is hormone production within your body. We already know from today's medical science that hormones act as catalysts in the body. When the hormone levels are high, we are more energized and cell replacement can occur faster and more smoothly. When hormone production is slow and its level is low, then the cell replacement is slower and we will age quickly. It is only in the last few years that scientists have discovered that by increasing the hormone levels in the body, we may be able to extend our lifespan significantly.[10]

Maintenance of hormone production in a healthy manner has also been a major concern in Chinese Qigong practice. According to Chinese medicine, glands that produce hormones were recognized since ancient times. The role of hormones was not understood. However, throughout a thousand years of practice and experience, Qigong practitioners understood that the essence of life is stored in the kidneys. Today, we know that this essence is actually the hormones produced from the adrenal glands on the top of the kidneys. The Chinese also believed that through stimulation of the testicles and ovaries, the life force could be increased. In addition, from still meditation practice, they learned how to lead the Qi to the brain and raise up the "spirit of vitality." It has also been found that through practice, bioelectricity can be led to the pituitary gland to stimulate growth hormone production. All of these practices are believed to be effective paths to longevity.

From medical science, we know that our hormone levels are significantly reduced when the last pieces of our bones are completed, between ages 29 to 30. Theoretically, when our body has completed constructing itself, it somehow triggers the reduction of our hormone levels. From this, you can see that maintaining the hormone levels in our body may be a key to longevity.

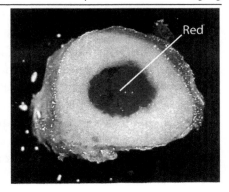

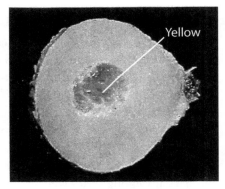

FIGURE 1-12. STRUCTURE OF A LONG BONE. RED BONE MARROW AND YELLOW BONE MARROW

Finally, in order to prevent ourselves from getting sick, we must also consider our immune system. According to Chinese medicine and Qigong, when Qi storage is abundant, you are sick less often. If we take a careful look, we can realize that every white blood cell is just like a fighting soldier. If we do not have enough Qi to supply them, their fighting capability will be low. It is just like a soldier who needs food to maintain his strength. When the Qi is strong, the immune system is strong. Therefore, the skin breathing technique was developed, that teaches a practitioner to lead the Qi to the surface of the skin to strengthen the "Guardian Qi" (Wei Qi, 衛氣) or an energetic component of the immune system near the skin surface.

Apart from the above required elements for your health and longevity, however, the most important thing you can do is to learn how to increase the quantity of Qi storage and how to consume it efficiently (i.e. quality of Qi's manifestation). Through a thousand years of study and practice, the Chinese have realized that in order to acquire these two important components of Qigong practice, you must understand and practice the method of "Embryonic Breathing" (Tai Xi, 胎息). Through this breathing, can raise up and concentrate your spirit to a high level, increase the quantity of your Qi and store it to an abundant level. If you are interested in this subject, please refer to the book: *Qigong Meditation—Embryonic Breathing*, by Dr. Yang, Jwing-Ming.

From the foregoing, hopefully I have offered you a challenge for profound thought and understanding. Although most of these conclusions are drawn from my personal research, further study and verification is still needed. I deeply believe that if we can all open our minds and share our opinions together, we will be able to make our lives healthier and more meaningful.

1-3. The History of Qigong 氣功簡史

The history of Chinese Qigong can be roughly divided into four periods. We know little about the first period, which is considered to have started when the *Yi Jing* (*Book of Changes*) (易經) was introduced sometime before 1122 B.C., and to have extended until the Han Dynasty (206 B.C., 漢朝) when Buddhism and its meditation methods were imported from India. This infusion brought Qigong practice and meditation into the second period, the religious Qigong era. This period lasted until the Liang Dynasty (502-557 A.D., 梁朝), when it was discovered that Qigong could be used for martial purposes. This was the beginning of the third period, that of martial Qigong. Many different martial Qigong styles were created based on the theories and principles of Buddhist and Daoist Qigong. This period lasted until the overthrow of the Qing Dynasty (清朝) in 1911; from that point Chinese Qigong training was mixed with Qigong practices from India, Japan, and many other countries.

Before the Han Dynasty (Before 206 B.C.) 漢前

The *Yi Jing* (*Book of Changes*; 1122 B.C.) was probably the first Chinese book related to Qi. It introduced the concept of the three natural energies or powers (San Cai, 三才): Tian (Heaven, 天), Di (Earth, 地), and Ren (Man, 人). Studying the relationship of these three natural powers was the first step in the development of Qigong.

From 1766-1154 B.C. (the Shang Dynasty, 商朝), the Chinese capital was located in today's An Yang in Henan province (河南，安陽). An archaeological dig, at a late Shang Dynasty burial ground called Yin Xu (殷墟) discovered more than 160,000 pieces of turtle shell and animal bone that were covered with written characters. This writing, called "Jia Gu Wen" (甲骨文) (Oracle-Bone Scripture), is the earliest evidence of the Chinese use of the written word. Most of the information recorded was of a religious nature. Together with these oracle-bone scriptures, the so called Bian Shi (砭石) (stone probes) (Figure 1-13) were discovered. The name Bian Shi was recorded in the *Nei Jing* (內經), which mentioned that during the reign of the Yellow Emperor (2690-2590 B.C.) (Huang Di, 黃帝) Bian Shi were already being used to adjust people's Qi circulation.

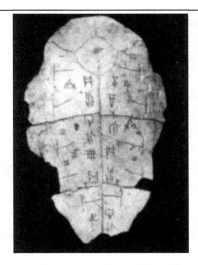 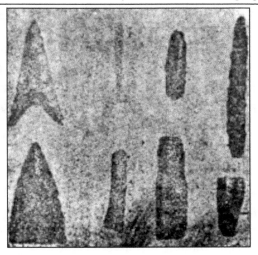

FIGURE 1-13. JIA GU WEN (ORACLE-BONE SCRIPTURE) AND BIAN SHI (STONE PROBES)

During the Zhou Dynasty (1122-934 B.C.) (周朝), Lao Zi (Li Er) (老子；李耳) mentioned certain breathing techniques in his classic *Dao De Jing* (or *Tao Te Ching*) (道德經) (*Classic on the Virtue of the Dao*). He stressed that the way to obtain health was to "concentrate on Qi and achieve softness" (Zhuan Qi Zhi Rou, 專氣致柔). Later, the *Shi Ji* (史紀) (*Historical Record*) from in the Spring and Autumn and Warring States Periods (770-221 B.C.) (Chun Qiu Zhan Guo, 春秋戰國) also described more complete methods of breath training. About 300 B.C., the Daoist philosopher Zhuang Zi (莊子) described the relationship between health and the breath in his book *Nan Hua Jing* (南華經). It states: "The real person's (i.e. immortal's) breathing reaches down to their heels. The normal person's breathing in the throat."[11] This suggests that a breathing method for Qi circulation was already being used by some Daoists at that time.

During the Qin and Han Dynasties (221 B.C.-220 A.D.) (秦，漢), there were several medical references to Qigong in the literature, such as the *Nan Jing* (*Classic on Disorders*) (難經) by the famous physician Bian Que (扁鵲), that describes how breathing was used to increase Qi circulation. *Jin Kui Yao Lue* (*Prescriptions from the Golden Chamber*) (金匱要略) by Zhang, Zhong-Jing (張仲景) discusses the use of breathing and acupuncture to maintain good Qi flow. *Zhou Yi Can Tong Qi* (*A Comparative Study of the Zhou (Dynasty) Book of Changes*) (周易參同契) by Wei, Bo-Yang (魏伯陽) explains the relationship of human beings to nature's forces and Qi. It can be seen from this list that up to this time, almost all of the Qigong publications were written by scholars such as Lao Zi (老子) and Zhuang Zi (莊子), or physicians such as Bian Que and Wei, Bo-Yang.

From the Han Dynasty to the Beginning of the Liang Dynasty
(206 B.C.-502 A.D.) 漢 - 梁

Because many Han emperors were intelligent and wise, the Han Dynasty was a glorious and peaceful period. It was during the Dong Han Dynasty (東漢) (c. 58 A.D.) (East Han Dynasty) that Buddhism was imported to China from India. The Han emperor became a sincere Buddhist; Buddhism soon spread and became very popular. Many Buddhist meditation and Qigong practices, which had been practiced in India for thousands of years, were absorbed into the Chinese culture. The Buddhist temples taught many Qigong practices, especially the still meditation of Chan (Ren) (禪，忍), which marked a new era of Chinese Qigong. Much of the deeper Qigong theory and practices which had been developed in India were brought to China. Unfortunately, since the training was directed at attaining Buddhahood, the training practices and theory were recorded in the Buddhist bibles and kept secret. For hundreds of years, the religious Qigong training was never taught to laymen. Only in last century has it been available to the general populace.

Not long after Buddhism had been imported into China, a Daoist by the name of Zhang, Dao-Ling (張道陵) combined the traditional Daoist principles with Buddhism and created a religion called Dao Jiao (道教). Many of its meditation methods were a combination of the principles and training methods of both sources.

Since Tibet had developed its own branch of Buddhism with its own training system and methods of attaining Buddhahood, Tibetan Buddhists were also invited to China to preach. In time, their practices were also absorbed.

It was in this period that the traditional Chinese Qigong practitioners finally had a chance to compare their arts with the religious Qigong practices imported mainly from India. While the scholarly and medical Qigong had been concerned with maintaining and improving health, the newly imported religious Qigong was concerned with far more. Contemporary documents and Qigong styles from that period show clearly that the religious practitioners trained their Qi to a much deeper level, worked with many internal functions of the body, and strove to obtain control of their bodies, minds, and spirits with the goal of escaping from the cycle of reincarnation.

While the Qigong practices and meditations were being passed down secretly within the monasteries, traditional scholars and physicians continued their Qigong research. During the Jin Dynasty (晉朝) in the third century A.D., a famous physician named Hua Tuo (華佗) used acupuncture for anesthesia in surgery. The Daoist Jun Qian (君倩) used the movements of animals to create the Wu Qin Xi (五禽戲) (Five Animal Sports), that taught people how to increase their Qi circulation through specific movements. Some say that the Wu Qin Xi was actually created by Hua Tuo. Also, in this period a physician named Ge Hong (葛洪) mentioned using the mind to lead and increase Qi in his book *Bao Pu Zi (Embracing Simplicity)* (抱朴子). Sometime in the period between 420 and 581 A.D. Tao, Hong-Jing (陶弘景) compiled the *Yang Shen Yan Ming Lu*

(*Records of Nourishing the Body and Extending Life*) (養身延命錄), which showed many Qigong techniques.

From the Liang Dynasty to the End of the Qing Dynasty (502-1911 A.D.) 梁 - 清

During the Liang Dynasty (梁朝) (502-557 A.D.), the emperor invited a Buddhist monk named Da Mo (達磨) (i.e. Bodhi-Dharma), who was once an Indian prince, to preach Buddhism in China. The emperor decided he did not like Da Mo's Buddhist theory, so the monk withdrew to the Shaolin Temple (少林寺). When Da Mo arrived, he saw that the priests were weak and sickly, so he shut himself away to ponder the problem. He emerged after nine years of seclusion and wrote two classics: *Yi Jin Jing* (*Muscle/Tendon Changing Classic*) (易筋經) and *Xi Sui Jing* (*Marrow/Brain Washing Classic*) (洗髓經). The *Muscle/Tendon Changing Classic* taught the priests how to gain health and change their physical bodies from weak to strong. The *Marrow/Brain Washing Classic* taught the priests how to use Qi to clean the bone marrow and strengthen the blood and immune system, as well as how to energize the brain and attain enlightenment. Because the *Marrow/Brain Washing Classic* was more difficult to understand and practice, the training methods were passed down secretly to only a very few disciples in each generation.

After the priests practiced the Muscle/Tendon Changing exercises, they found that not only did they improve their health, but they also greatly increased their strength. When this training was integrated into the martial arts forms, it increased the effectiveness of their techniques. In addition to this martial Qigong training, the Shaolin priests also created five animal styles of Gongfu that imitated the way different animals fight. The animals imitated were the tiger, leopard, dragon, snake, and crane.

Outside of the monastery, the development of Qigong continued during the Sui and Tang Dynasties (隋，唐) (581-907 A.D.). Chao, Yuan-Fang (巢元方) compiled the *Zhu Bing Yuan Hou Lun* (*Thesis on the Origins and Symptoms of Various Diseases*) (諸病源候論), which is a veritable encyclopedia of Qigong methods, listing 260 different ways of increasing the Qi flow. The *Qian Jin Fang* (*Thousand Gold Prescriptions*) (千金方) by Sun, Si-Miao (孫思邈) described the method of leading Qi, and also described the use of the Six Sounds. The Buddhists and Daoists had already been using the Six Sounds to regulate Qi in the internal organs for some time. Sun Si-Miao also introduced a massage system called Lao Zi's 49 Massage Techniques. *Wai Tai Mi Yao* (*The Extra Important Secret*) (外台祕要) by Wang Tao (王燾) discussed the use of breathing and herbal therapies for disorders of Qi circulation.

During the Song, Jin, and Yuan Dynasties (宋，金，元) (960-1368 A.D.), *Yang Shen Jue* (*Life Nourishing Secrets*) (養生訣) by Zhang, An-Dao (張安道) discussed several Qigong practices. *Ru Men Shi Shi* (*The Confucian Point of View*) (儒門視事) by Zhang, Zi-He (張子和) describes the use of Qigong to cure external injuries such as cuts and sprains. *Lan Shi Mi Cang* (*Secret Library of the Orchid Room*) (蘭室祕藏) by Li Guo (李果) describes the use of Qigong and herbal remedies for internal disorders. *Ge Zhi Yu Lun* (*A Further Thesis of Complete Study*) (格致餘論) by Zhu, Dan-Xi (朱丹溪) provided a theoretical explanation for the use of Qigong in curing disease.

During the Song Dynasty (宋朝) (960-1279 A.D.), Zhang, San-Feng (張三豐) is believed to have created Taijiquan (or Tai Chi Chuan) (太極拳). Taiji followed a different approach in its use of Qigong than did Shaolin. While Shaolin emphasized Wai Dan (外丹) (External Elixir) Qigong exercises, Taiji emphasized Nei Dan (內丹) (Internal Elixir) Qigong training.

In 1026 A.D., the famous brass man of acupuncture was designed and built by Dr. Wang, Wei-Yi (王唯一). Before that time, the many publications that discussed acupuncture theory, principles, and treatment techniques disagreed with each other and left many points unclear. When Dr. Wang built his brass man, he also wrote a book called *Tong Ren Yu Xue Zhen Jiu Tu* (*Illustration of the Brass Man Acupuncture and Moxibustion*) (銅人俞穴鍼灸圖). He explained the relationship of the 12 organs and the 12 Qi channels, clarified many of the points of confusion, and, for the first time, systematically organized acupuncture theory and principles.

In 1034 A.D., Dr. Wang used acupuncture to cure the emperor Ren Zong (仁宗). With the support of the emperor, acupuncture flourished. In order to encourage acupuncture medical research, the emperor built a temple to Bian Que, who wrote the Nan Jing, and worshiped him as the ancestor of acupuncture. Acupuncture technology developed so much that even the Jin people in the distant North requested the brass man and other acupuncture technology as a condition for peace. Between 1102 to 1106 A.D., Dr. Wang dissected the bodies of prisoners and added more information to the Nan Jing. His work contributed greatly to the advancement of Qigong and Chinese medicine by giving a clear and systematic idea of the circulation of Qi in the human body.

Later, in the Southern Song Dynasty (南宋) (1127-1279 A.D.), Marshal Yue Fei (岳飛) was credited with creating several internal Qigong exercises and martial arts. It is said that he created Ba Duan Jin (*The Eight Pieces of Brocade*) (八段錦) to improve the health of his soldiers. He is also known as the creator of the internal martial style Xingyi (形意). Eagle-style martial artists also claim that Yue Fei was the creator of their style.

From then until the end of the Qing Dynasty (清朝) (1911 A.D,), many other Qigong styles were founded. The well known ones include Hu Bu Gong (Tiger Step Gong) (虎步功), Shi Er Zhuang (Twelve Postures) (十二庄), and Jiao Hua Gong (Beggar Gong) (叫化功). Also in this period, many documents related to Qigong were published, such as *Bao Shen Mi Yao* (*The Secret Important Document of Body Protection*) (保身祕要) by Cao, Yuan-Bai (曹元白), which described moving and stationary Qigong practices; and *Yang Shen Fu Yu* (*Brief Introduction to Nourishing the Body*) (養生膚語) by Chen, Ji-Ru (陳繼儒), about the three treasures: Jing (精) (essence), Qi (氣) (internal energy), and Shen (神) (spirit). Also, *Yi Fan Ji Jie* (*The Total Introduction to Medical Prescriptions*) (醫方集介) by Wang, Fan-An (汪汎庵) reviewed and summarized the previously published materials; and *Nei Gong Tu Shuo* (*Illustrated Explanation of Nei Gong*) (內功圖說) by Wang, Zu-Yuan (王祖源) presented the Twelve Pieces of Brocade and explained the idea of combining both moving and stationary Qigong.

In the late Ming Dynasty (明朝) (around 1640 A.D.), a martial Qigong style, Huo Long Gong (火龍功) (Fire Dragon Gong), was created by the Taiyang martial stylists (太陽宗). The well-known internal martial art style Baguazhang (八卦掌) (Eight Trigrams Palm) is believed to have been created by Dong, Hai-Chuan (董海川) late in the Qing Dynasty (清朝) (1644-1911 A.D.). This style is now gaining in popularity throughout the world.

During the Qing Dynasty, Tibetan meditation and martial techniques became widespread in China for the first time. This was due to the encouragement and interest of the Manchurian emperors in the royal palace, as well as others of high rank in society.

From the End of Qing Dynasty to the Present 清後

Before 1911 A.D., Chinese society was still very conservative and old-fashioned. Even though China had been expanding its contact with the outside world for the previous hundred years, the outside world had little influence beyond the coastal regions. With the overthrow of the Qing Dynasty in 1911 and the founding of the Chinese Republic, the nation began changing as never before. Since this time Qigong practice has entered a new era. Because of the ease of communication in the modern world, Western culture now has great influence on the Orient. Many Chinese have opened their minds and changed their traditional ideas, especially in Taiwan and Hong Kong. Various Qigong styles are now being taught openly, and many formerly secret documents have been published. Modern methods of communication have opened up Qigong to a much wider audience than ever before, and people now have the opportunity to study and understand many different styles. In addition, people are now able to compare Chinese Qigong to similar arts from other countries such as India, Japan, Korea, and the Middle East.

I believe that in the near future, Qigong will be considered the most exciting and challenging field of research. It is an ancient science just waiting to be investigated with the help of the new technologies now being developed at an almost explosive rate. Anything we can do to speed up this research will greatly help humanity to understand and improve itself.

1-4. CATEGORIES OF QIGONG 氣功之分類

Often, people ask me the same question: Is jogging, weight lifting, or dancing a kind of Qigong practice? To answer this question, let us trace back Qigong history to before the Chinese Qin and Han Dynastic periods (秦，漢) (255 B.C.-223 A.D.). Then you can see that the origins of many Qigong practices were actually in dancing. Through dancing, the physical body was exercised and the health of the physical body was maintained. Also, through dancing and matching movements with music, the mind was regulated

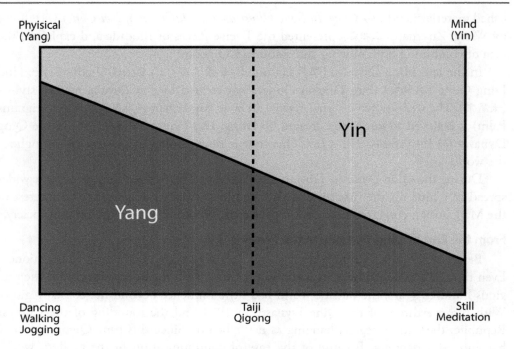

Phyisical
(Yang)

Mind
(Yin)

Yin

Yang

Dancing
Walking
Jogging

Taiji
Qigong

Still
Meditation

FIGURE 1-14. THE RANGE OF DEFINED QIGONG

into a harmonious state. From this harmonious mind, the spirit can be raised to a more energized state or can be calmed down to a peaceful level. This Qigong dancing later passed to Japan during the Chinese Han Dynasty, and became a very elegant, slow, and high style of dancing in the Japanese royal court. This Taijiquan-like dancing is still practiced in Japan today.

The ways of African or Native American dancing in which the body is bounced up and down is also known as a means of loosening up the joints and improving Qi circulation. Naturally, jogging, weight lifting, or even walking are a kind of Qigong practice. Therefore, we can say that any activity which is able to regulate the Qi circulation in the body is a Qigong practice.

Let us define it more clearly. In Figure 1-14, if the left vertical line represents the amount of usage of the physical body (Yang, 陽), and the right vertical line is the usage of the mind (Yin, 陰), then we can see that the more you practice toward the left, the more physical effort, and the less mind, is needed. The activity can be aerobic dancing, walking, or jogging in which the mind usage is relatively small compared to physical action. In this kind of Qigong practice, normally you do not need special training, and it is classified as layman Qigong. In the middle point, the mind and the physical activity are almost equally important. This kind of Qigong will be the slow moving Qigong commonly practiced, in which the mind is used to lead the Qi in coordination with the movements. Examples are Taiji Qigong, The Eight Pieces of Brocade, The Five Animal Sports, and many others are very typical Qigong exercises, especially in Chinese medical and martial arts societies.

However, when you reach a profound level of Qigong practice, the mind becomes more critical and important. When you reach this high level, you are dealing with your mind while you are sitting still. Most of this mental Qigong training was practiced by the scholars and religious Qigong practitioners. In this practice, you may have a little physical movement in the lower abdomen. However, the main focus of this Qigong practice lies in the peaceful mind or spiritual enlightenment that originates from the cultivation of your mind. This kind of Qigong practice includes Sitting Chan (Ren) (Zuo Chan, Ren; 坐禪，忍), Small Circulation Meditation (Xiao Zhou Tian, 小周天), Grand Circulation Meditation (Da Zhou Tian, 大周天), or Brain Washing Enlightenment Meditation (Xi Sui Gong, 洗髓功).

Theoretically speaking, in order to have good health, you will need to maintain your physical condition and also build up abundant Qi in your body. The best Qigong for health is actually located in the middle of our model, where you learn how to regulate your physical body and also your mind. From this Yin and Yang practice, your Qi can be circulated smoothly in the body.

Let us now review the traditional concepts of how Qigong was categorized. Generally speaking, all Qigong practices can be divided on the basis of their training theory and methods into two general categories: Wai Dan (外丹) (External Elixir) and Nei Dan (內丹) (Internal Elixir). Understanding the differences between them will give you a broader understanding of most Chinese Qigong practice.

External and Internal Elixirs (Wai Dan, Nei Dan; 外丹，內丹)

A. Wai Dan (External Elixir) 外丹

"Wai" (外) means "external" or "outside," and "Dan" (丹) means "elixir." External here means the skin surface of the body or the limbs, as opposed to the torso or the center of the body, which includes all of the vital organs. Elixir is a hypothetical, life-prolonging substance for which Chinese Daoists have been searching for several millennia. They originally thought that the elixir was something physical which could be prepared from herbs or chemicals purified in a furnace. After thousands of years of study and experimentation, they found that the elixir dwells in the body. In other words, if you want to prolong your life, you must find the elixir in your body, and then learn to cultivate, protect, and nourish it. Actually, the elixir is what we have understood the inner energy or Qi circulating in the body to be.

There are many ways of producing elixir or Qi in the body. For example, in Wai Dan Qigong practice, you may exercise your limbs by dancing or even walking. As you exercise, the Qi builds up in your arms and legs. When the Qi potential in your limbs builds to a high enough level, the Qi will flow through the channels, clearing any obstructions and flowing into the center of the body to nourish the organs. This is the main reason that a person who works out, or has a physical job is, generally healthier than someone who sits around all day.

Naturally, you may simply massage your body to produce the Qi. Through massage, you may stimulate the cells of your body to a higher energized state and therefore the Qi concentration will be raised and the circulation enhanced. Then, after massage you relax, and the higher levels of Qi on the skin surface and muscles will flow into the center of the body and thereby improve the Qi circulatory conditions in your internal organs. This is the theoretical foundation of the Tui Na Qigong massage (推拿) (pushing and grabbing massage).

Through acupuncture, you may also bring the Qi level near the skin surface to a higher level and from this stimulation, the Qi condition of the internal organs can be regulated through Qi channels. Therefore, acupuncture can also be classified as Wai Dan Qigong practice. Naturally, the herbal treatments are a way of Wai Dan practice as well.

From this, we can briefly conclude that any possible stimulation or exercise that accumulate a high level of Qi on the surface of the body, and then flow inward toward the center of the body, can be classified as Wai Dan (external elixir) (Figure 1-15).

B. Nei Dan (Internal Elixir) 內丹

"Nei" means "internal" and "Dan" again means "elixir." Thus, Nei Dan means to build the elixir internally. Here, internally means in the body instead of in the limbs. Normally, the Qi is built on the Qi vessels instead of the primary Qi channels. Whereas in Wai Dan the Qi is built up in the limbs or skin surface and then moved into the body through primary Qi channels, Nei Dan exercises build up Qi in the body and lead it out to the limbs (Figure 1-16).

Generally, speaking, Nei Dan theory is deeper than Wai Dan theory, and it is more difficult to understand and practice. Traditionally, most of the Nei Dan Qigong practices have been passed down more secretly than those of the Wai Dan. This is especially true of the highest levels of Nei Dan, such as Marrow/Brain Washing, which were passed down to only a few trusted disciples.

Schools of Qigong Practice 不同氣功流派

We can also classify Qigong into four major categories according to the purpose or final goal of the training: A. maintaining health; B. curing sickness; C. martial arts; D. enlightenment or Buddhahood. This is only a rough breakdown, however, since almost every style of Qigong serves more than one of the above purposes. For example, although martial Qigong focuses on increasing fighting effectiveness, it can also improve your health. Daoist Qigong aims for longevity and enlightenment, but to reach this goal you need to be in good health and know how to cure sickness. Because of this multi-purpose aspect of the categories, it will be simpler to discuss their backgrounds rather than the goals of their training. Knowing the history and basic principles of each category will help you to understand their Qigong more clearly.

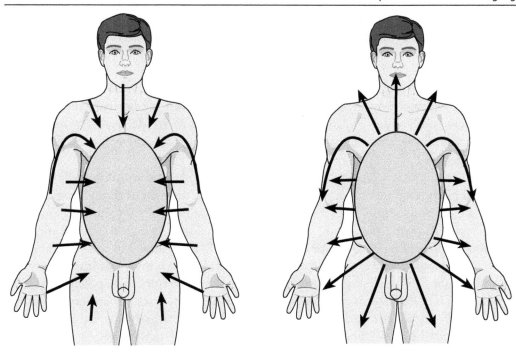

FIGURE 1-15. EXTERNAL ELIXIR (WAI DAN)　　　　FIGURE 1-16. INTERNAL ELIXIR (NEI DAN)

A. Scholar Qigong—for Maintaining Health 學者氣功－保身

In China before the Han Dynasty, there were two major schools of scholarship. One of them was created by Confucius (551-479 B.C.) (Kong Zi, 孔子) during the Spring and Autumn period. Later, his philosophy was popularized and enlarged by Mencius (372-289 B.C.) (Meng Zi, 孟子) in the Warring States Period. The scholars who practice his philosophy are commonly called Confucians or Confucianists (Ru Jia, 儒家). The key words to their basic philosophy are Loyalty (Zhong, 忠), Filial Piety (Xiao, 孝), Humanity (Ren, 仁), Kindness (Ai, 愛), Trust (Xin, 信), Justice (Yi, 義), Harmony (He, 和), and Peace (Ping, 平). Humanity and human feelings are the main subjects of study. Ru Jia philosophy has become the center of much of Chinese culture.

The second major school of scholarship was called Dao Jia (Daoism) (道家) and was created by Lao Zi (老子) in the 6th century B.C. Lao Zi is considered to be the author of a book called the *Dao De Jing* (*Classic on the Virtue of the Dao*) (道德經) which describes human morality. Later, in the Warring States Period, his follower Zhuang Zhou (莊周) wrote a book called *Zhuang Zi* (莊子) which led to the forming of another strong branch of Daoism. Before the Han Dynasty, Daoism was considered a branch of scholarship. However, in the Han Dynasty, traditional Daoism was combined with the Buddhism imported from India by Zhang, Dao-Ling (張道陵), and it began gradually to be treated as a religion. Therefore, the Daoism before the Han Dynasty should be considered scholarly Daoism rather than religious.

With regard to their contribution to Qigong, both schools emphasized maintaining health and preventing disease. They believed that many illnesses are caused by mental and emotional excesses. When a person's mind is not calm, balanced, and peaceful, the organs will not function normally. For example, depression can cause stomach ulcers and indigestion. Anger will cause the liver to malfunction. Sadness will cause stagnation and tightness in the lungs, and fear can disturb the normal functioning of the kidneys and bladder. They realized that if you want to avoid illness, you must learn to balance and relax your thoughts and emotions. This is called "regulating the mind" (Tiao Xin, 調心).

Therefore, the scholars emphasize gaining a peaceful mind through meditation. In their still meditation, the main part of the training is getting rid of thoughts so that the mind is clear and calm. When you become calm, the flow of thoughts and emotions slows down, and you feel mentally and emotionally neutral. This kind of meditation can be thought of as practicing emotional self-control. When you are in this "no thought" state, you become very relaxed, and can even relax deep down into your internal organs. When your body is this relaxed, your Qi will naturally flow smoothly and strongly. This kind of still meditation was very common in ancient Chinese scholar society.

In order to reach the goal of a calm and peaceful mind, the scholar's training focused on regulating the mind, body, and breath. They believed that as long as these three things were regulated, the Qi flow would be smooth and sickness would not occur. This is why the Qi training of the scholars is called "Xiu Qi" (修氣), which means "cultivating Qi." "Xiu" (修) in Chinese means to regulate, to cultivate, or to repair. It also means to maintain in good condition. This is very different from the religious Daoist Qi training after the Han Dynasty which was called "Lian Qi" (練氣), translated as "train Qi." "Lian" (練) meaning to drill or to practice to make stronger.

Many of the Qigong documents written by the Confucians and Daoists were limited to the maintenance of health. The scholar's attitude in Qigong was to follow his natural destiny and maintain his health. This philosophy is quite different from that of the religious Daoist after the Han Dynasty, who believed that one's destiny could be changed. They believed that it is possible to train your Qi to make it stronger; and to extend your life. It is said in scholarly society: "in human life, seventy is rare."[12] You should understand that few of the common people in ancient times lived past seventy because of the lack of good food and modern medical technology. It is also said: "peace with Heaven and delight in your destiny" (An Tian Le Ming, 安天樂命); and "cultivate the body and await destiny" (Xiu Shen Si Ming, 修身俟命). Compare this with the philosophy of the later Daoists, who said: "one hundred and twenty means dying young."[13] They believed and have proven that human life can be lengthened and destiny can be resisted and overcome.

Confucianism and Daoism were the two major scholarly schools in China, but there were many other schools which were also more or less involved in Qigong practices. We will not discuss them here because there is only a very limited number of Qigong documents from these schools.

B. Medical Qigong—for Healing 醫療氣功－治病

In ancient Chinese society, most emperors respected the scholars and were influenced by their philosophy. Doctors were not regarded highly because they made their diagnosis by touching the patient's body, which was considered characteristic of the lower classes in society. Although the doctors developed a profound and successful medical science, they were commonly looked down on by others. However, they continued to work hard and study, and quietly passed down the results of their research to subsequent generations.

Of all the groups studying Qigong in China, the doctors have been working at it the longest. Since the discovery of Qi circulation in the human body about four thousand years ago, the Chinese doctors have devoted a major portion of their efforts to studying the behavior of Qi. Their efforts resulted in acupuncture, acupressure or Cavity Press massage, and herbal treatment.

In addition, many Chinese doctors used their medical knowledge to create different sets of Qigong exercises either for maintaining health or for curing specific illnesses. Chinese medical doctors believed that doing only sitting or still meditation to regulate the body, mind, and breathing as the scholars did was not enough to cure sickness. They believed that in order to increase the Qi circulation, you must move. Although a calm and peaceful mind was important for health, exercising the body was more important. They learned through their medical practice that people who exercised properly became sick less often, and their bodies degenerated less quickly than was the case with people who just sat around. They also realized that specific body movements could increase the Qi circulation in specific organs. They reasoned from this that such exercises could also be used to treat specific illnesses and to restore the normal functioning of these organs.

Some of these movements are similar to the way in that certain animals move. It is clear that in order for an animal to survive in the wild, it must have an instinct for how to protect its body. Part of this instinct involves building up its Qi, and keeping its Qi from being lost. We humans have lost many of these instincts over the years that we have been separating ourselves from nature.

Many doctors developed Qigong exercises that were modeled after animal movements to maintain health and cure sickness. A typical, well known set of such exercises is "Wu Qin Xi" (Five Animal Sports) (五禽戲) created by Dr. Jun Qing (君倩) (Note: Some documents credit Dr. Hua Tuo (華佗) as the creator of Wu Qin Xi.) Another famous set based on similar principles is called "Ba Duan Jin" (The Eight Pieces of Brocade) (八段錦). It was created by Marshal Yue Fei (岳飛) who, interestingly enough, was a soldier rather than a doctor.

In addition, using their medical knowledge of Qi circulation, Chinese doctors used their research until they found the specific movements could help cure particular illnesses and health problems. Not surprisingly, many of these movements were not unlike the ones used to maintain health, since many illnesses are caused by unbalanced Qi. When an imbalance continues for a long period of time, the organs will be affected, and may be physically damaged. It is just like running a machine without supplying the proper electrical current—over time, the machine will be damaged. Chinese doctors believe that before physical damage to an organ shows up in a patient's body, there is first an abnormality in the Qi balance and circulation. Abnormal Qi circulation occurs at the very beginning of illness and organ damage. When Qi is too positive (Yang) or too negative (Yin) in a specific organ's Qi channel, your physical organ is beginning to suffer damage. If you do not correct the Qi circulation, that organ will malfunction or degenerate. The best way to heal someone is to adjust and balance the Qi even before there is any physical problem. Therefore, correcting or increasing the normal Qi circulation is the major goal of acupuncture or acupressure treatments. Herbs and special diets are also considered important treatments in regulating the Qi in the body.

As long as the illness is limited to the level of Qi stagnation and there is no physical organ damage, the Qigong exercises used for maintaining health can be used to readjust the Qi circulation and treat the problem. However, if the sickness is already so serious that the physical organs have started to fail, then the situation has become critical and a specific treatment is necessary. The treatment can involve acupuncture, herbs, or even an operation, as well as specific Qigong exercises designed to speed up the healing or even to cure the sickness. For example, ulcers and asthma can often be cured or helped by some simple exercises. Recently in both mainland China and Taiwan, certain Qigong exercises have been shown to be effective in treating certain kinds of cancer.

Over the thousands of years of observing nature and themselves, some Qigong practitioners went even deeper. They realized that the body's Qi circulation changes with the seasons, and that it is a good idea to help the body out during these periodic adjustments. They noticed also that in each season different organs have characteristic problems. For example, in the beginning of Fall, the lungs have to adapt to the colder air that you are breathing. While this adjustment is going on, the lungs are susceptible to disturbance, so your lungs may feel uncomfortable and you may catch colds easily. Your digestive system is also affected during seasonal changes. Your appetite may increase, or you may have diarrhea. When the temperature goes down, your kidneys and bladder will start to give you trouble. For example, because the kidneys are stressed, you may feel pain in the back. Focusing on these seasonal Qi disorders, the meditators created a set of movements which can be used to speed up the body's adjustment.

In addition to Marshal Yue Fei, many people were not doctors also created sets of medical Qigong. These sets were probably originally created to maintain health, and later were also used for curing sickness.

C. Martial Qigong—for Fighting 武學氣功－防身

Chinese martial Qigong was probably not developed until Da Mo (達磨) wrote the *Muscle/Tendon Changing and Marrow/Brain Washing Classic* (*Yi Jin Jing, Xi Sui Jing*, 易筋經‧洗髓經) in the Shaolin Temple (少林寺) during the Liang Dynasty (502-557 A.D.) (梁朝). When Shaolin monks trained in Da Mo's Muscle/Tendon Changing Qigong, they found that they could not only improve their health but also greatly increase the power of their martial techniques. Since then, many martial styles have developed Qigong sets to increase their effectiveness. In addition, many martial styles have been created based on Qigong theory. Martial artists have played a major role in Chinese Qigong society.

When Qigong theory was first applied to the martial arts, it was used to increase the power and efficiency of the muscles. The theory is very simple—the mind (Yi, 意) is used to lead Qi to the muscles to energize them so that they function more efficiently. The average person generally uses his muscles at about 40% maximum efficiency. If one can train his concentration and use his strong Yi (the mind generated from clear thinking) to lead Qi to the muscles effectively, he will be able to energize the muscles to a higher level and, therefore, increase his fighting effectiveness.

As acupuncture theory became better understood, fighting techniques were able to reach even more advanced levels. Martial artists learned to attack specific areas, such as vital acupuncture cavities, to disturb the enemy's Qi flow, and create imbalances that caused injury or even death. In order to do this, the practitioner must understand the route and timing of the Qi circulation in the human body. He also has to train so that he can strike the cavities accurately and to the correct depth. These cavity strike techniques are called "Dian Xue" (點穴) (Pointing Cavities) or "Dian Mai" (點脈) (Pointing Vessels).

Most of the martial Qigong practices help to improve the practitioner's health. However, there are other martial Qigong practices which, although they build up some special skill which is useful for fighting, also damage the practitioner's health. An example of this is Iron Sand Palm (Tie Sha Zhang, 鐵砂掌). Although this training can build up amazing destructive power, it can also harm your hands and affect the Qi circulation in the hands and internal organs.

As mentioned in Chapter 1, since the sixth century, many martial styles have been created that were based on Qigong theory. They can be roughly divided into external and internal styles.

The external styles emphasize building Qi in the limbs to coordinate with the physical martial techniques. They follow the theory of Wai Dan (外丹) (External Elixir) Qigong, which usually generates Qi in the limbs through special exercises. The concentrated mind is used during the exercises to energize the Qi. This increases muscular strength significantly, and therefore increases the effectiveness of the martial techniques. Qigong can also be used to train the body to resist punches and kicks. In this training,

Qi is led to energize the skin and the muscles, enabling them to resist a blow without injury. This training is commonly called "Iron Shirt" (Tie Bu Shan, 鐵布衫) or "Golden Bell Cover" (Jin Zhong Zhao, 金鐘罩). The martial styles that use Wai Dan Qigong training are normally called external styles (Wai Jia, 外家) or Hard Qigong training is called Hard Gong (Ying Gong, 硬功). Shaolin Gongfu is a typical example of a style that uses Wai Dan martial Qigong.

Although Wai Dan Qigong can help the martial artist increase his power, there is a disadvantage. Because Wai Dan Qigong emphasizes training the external muscles, it can cause overdevelopment. This can cause a problem called "energy dispersion" (San Gong, 散功) when the practitioner gets older. In order to remedy this, when an external martial artist reaches a high level of external Qigong training he will start training internal Qigong, which specializes in curing the energy dispersion problem. That is why it is said: "Shaolin Gongfu from external to internal."

Internal Martial Qigong is based on the theory of Nei Dan (Internal Elixir). In this method, Qi is generated in the body instead of the limbs, and this Qi is then led to the limbs to increase power. In order to lead Qi to the limbs, the techniques must be soft and muscle usage must be kept to a minimum. The training and theory of Nei Dan martial Qigong is much more difficult than those of Wai Dan martial Qigong. Interested readers should refer to the author's book: *Tai Chi Theory and Martial Power*.

Several internal martial styles were created in the Wudang (武當山) and Emei Mountains (峨嵋山). Popular styles are Taijiquan, Baguazhang, Liu He Ba Fa, and Xingyiquan. However, you should understand that even the internal martial styles, which are commonly called Soft Styles, must on some occasions use muscular strength while fighting. That means in order to have strong power in the fight, the Qi must be led to the muscular body and manifested externally. Therefore, once an internal martial artist has achieved a degree of competence in internal Qigong, he or she should also learn how to use harder, more external techniques. That is why it is said: "The internal styles are from soft to hard."

In the last fifty years, some of the Taiji Qigong or Taijiquan practitioners have developed training aimed mainly for health, and is called "Wuji Qigong" (無極氣功), which means "no extremities Qigong." Wuji is the state of neutrality which precedes Taiji, that is the state of relative, complimentary opposites. When there are thoughts and feeling in your mind, there is Yin and Yang, but if you can still your mind you can return to the emptiness of Wuji. When you achieve this state your mind is centered and clear, your body relaxed, and your Qi is able to flow naturally and smoothly to reach the proper balance by itself. Wuji Qigong has become very popular in many parts of China, especially Shanghai and Canton.

You can see that, although Qigong is widely studied in Chinese martial arts, the main focus of training was originally placed on increasing fighting ability rather than health. Good health was considered a by-product of training. It was not until this century that the health aspect of martial Qigong started receiving greater attention. This is especially true in the internal martial arts.

D. Religious Qigong—for Enlightenment or Buddhahood 宗教氣功－成仙立佛

Religious Qigong, though not as popular as other categories in China, is recognized as having achieved the highest accomplishments of all the Qigong categories. It used to be kept secret by the monastic society, and it is only in this century that it has been revealed to laymen.

In China, religious Qigong includes mainly Daoist and Buddhist Qigong. The main purpose of their training is striving for enlightenment, or what the Buddhists refer to as Buddhahood. They are looking for a way to lift themselves above normal human suffering, and to escape from the cycle of continual reincarnation. They believe that all human suffering is caused by the seven emotions and six desires (Qi Qing Liu Yu, 七情六慾). The seven emotions are happiness (Xi, 喜), anger (Nu, 怒), sorrow (Ai, 哀), joy (Le, 樂), love (Ai, 愛), hate (Hen, 恨), and desire (Yu, 慾). The six desires are the six sensory pleasures derived from the eyes, ears, nose, tongue, body, and mind. If you are still bound to these emotions and desires, you will reincarnate after your death. To avoid reincarnation, you must train your spirit to reach a very high stage where it is strong enough to be independent after your death. This spirit will enter the heavenly kingdom and gain eternal peace. This training is hard to do in the everyday world, so practitioners frequently flee society and move into the solitude of the mountains where they can concentrate all of their energies on self-cultivation.

Religious Qigong practitioners train to strengthen their internal Qi to nourish their spirit (Shen) until the spirit is able to survive the death of the physical body. Marrow/Brain Washing Qigong training is necessary to reach this stage. It enables them to lead Qi to the forehead, where the spirit resides, and raise the brain to a higher energy state. This training used to be restricted to only a few priests who had reached an advanced level. Tibetan Buddhists were also involved heavily in this training. Over the last two thousand years, the Tibetan Buddhists, the Chinese Buddhists, and the Daoists have followed the same principles to become the three major religious schools of Qigong training.

This religious striving toward enlightenment or Buddhahood is recognized as the highest and most difficult level of Qigong. Many Qigong practitioners reject the rigors of this religious striving, and practice Marrow/Brain Washing Qigong solely for the purpose of longevity. It was these people who eventually revealed the secrets of Marrow/Brain Washing to the outside world. If you are interested in knowing more about this training, you may refer to: *Qigong—The Secret of Youth,* by this author.

From the above brief summary, you may obtain a general idea of how Chinese Qigong can be categorized. From the understanding of this general concept, you should not have further doubts about any Qigong you are training.

In the next section, we will discuss general Qigong training theory. This theoretical discussion of Qigong practice will offer you a foundation upon which to build your training. Without this scientific theoretical support, your mind will continue wondering and wandering. Understanding the theory is like learning how to read a map, which can direct you to the final goal of practice without confusion.

1-5. Qigong Training Theory 氣功練習之理論

Many people think that Qigong is a difficult subject to comprehend. In some ways, this is true. However, you must understand one thing: regardless of how difficult the Qigong theory and practice of a particular style is, the basic theory and principles are very simple and remain the same for all Qigong styles. The basic theory and principles form the root of the entire Qigong practice. If you understand these roots, you will be able to grasp the key to the practice and grow. All of the Qigong styles originated from these roots, but each one has blossomed differently.

In this section, we will discuss these basic Qigong training theories and principles. With this knowledge as foundation, you will be able to understand not only what you should be doing, but also why you are doing it. Naturally, it is impossible to discuss all of the basic Qigong ideas in such a short section. However, it will offer you the key to open the gate into the spacious, four thousand year old garden of Chinese Qigong. If you wish to know more about the theory of Qigong, please refer to *The Root of Chinese Qigong,* by this author.

The Concept of Yin and Yang, Kan and Li 陰陽坎離之概念

The concept of Yin (陰) and Yang (陽) is the foundation of Chinese philosophy. From this philosophy, Chinese culture was developed. Naturally, this includes Chinese medicine and Qigong practice. Therefore, in order to understand Qigong, first you should study the concept of Yin and Yang. In addition, you should also understand the concept of Kan (坎) and Li (離) which, unfortunately, has been commonly confused with the concept of Yin and Yang even in China.

The Chinese have long believed that the universe is made up of two opposite forces—Yin (陰) and Yang (陽)—which must balance each other. When these two forces begin to lose their balance, nature finds a way to rebalance them. If the imbalance is significant, disaster will occur. However, when these two forces interact with each other smoothly and harmoniously, they manifest power and generate the millions of living beings.

As mentioned earlier, Yin and Yang theory is also applied to the three great natural powers: heaven (Tian, 天), earth (Di, 地), and man (Ren, 人). For example, if the Yin and Yang forces of heaven (i.e. energy which comes to us from the sky) lose their balance, there can be tornadoes, hurricanes, or other natural disasters. When the Yin and Yang forces lose their balance on earth, rivers can change their paths and earthquakes can occur. When the Yin and Yang forces in the human body lose their balance, sickness and even death can occur. Experience has shown that the Yin and Yang balance in man is affected by the Yin and Yang balances of the earth and heaven. Similarly, the Yin and Yang balance of the earth is influenced by the heaven's Yin and Yang. Therefore, if you wish to have a healthy body and live a long life, you need to know how to adjust your body's Yin and Yang, and how to coordinate your Qi with the Yin and Yang energy of heaven and earth. The study of Yin and Yang in the human body is the root of Chinese medicine and Qigong.

Furthermore, the Chinese have also classified everything in the universe according to Yin and Yang. Even feelings, thoughts, strategy and the spirit are covered. For example, female is Yin and male is Yang, night is Yin and day is Yang, weak is Yin and strong is Yang, backward is Yin and forward is Yang, sad is Yin and happy is Yang, defense is Yin and offense is Yang, and so on.

Practitioners of Chinese medicine and Qigong believe that they must seek to understand the Yin and Yang of nature and the human body before they can adjust and regulate the body's energy balance into a more harmonious state. Only then can health be maintained and the causes of sicknesses be corrected.

Something else you should understand is that the concept of Yin and Yang is relative instead of absolute. For example, the number seven is Yang compared with three. However, if seven is compared with ten, then it is Yin. That means in order to decide Yin or Yang, a reference point must first be chosen. Therefore, if five is the Yin and Yang balance number, then seven is Yang and three is Yin. If we choose zero as the Yin and Yang balance number, then any positive is Yang and any negative number is Yin.

However, if what we are interested in is the most negative number, then we may choose the negative number as Yang and positive number as Yin with zero as the central number. For example, generally speaking in Qigong, techniques that can be seen physically and are the manifestation of Qi are considered Yang, and the techniques that cannot be seen but felt are created as Yin. When the Yin and Yang concept is applied in Chinese medicine, since the Qi is the major concern and plays the main role in medicine, it is considered Yang, while the blood (physical) is considered Yin.

Now let us discuss how the concept of Yin and Yang is applied to the Qi circulating in the human body. Many people, even some Qigong practitioners, are still confused by this. When it is said that Qi can be either Yin or Yang, it does not mean that there are two different kinds of Qi like male and female, fire and water, or positive and negative charges. Qi is energy, and energy itself does not have Yin and Yang. It is like the energy that is generated from the sparking of negative and positive charges. Charges have the potential for generating energy, but are not the energy itself.

When it is said that Qi is Yin or Yang, it means that the Qi is too strong or too weak for a particular circumstance. Again, this is relative and not absolute. Naturally, this implies that the potential that generates the Qi is strong or weak. For example, the Qi from the sun is Yang Qi, and Qi from the moon is Yin Qi, because the sun's energy is

Yang in comparison to Human Qi, while the moon's is Yin. In any discussion of energy where people are involved, Human Qi is used as the standard. People are always especially interested in what concerns them directly, so it is natural that we are interested primarily in Human Qi and tend to view all Qi from the perspective of Human Qi. This is not unlike looking at the universe from the physical perspective of the Earth.

When we look at the Yin and Yang of Qi within the human body, however, we must redefine our point of reference. For example, when a person is dead, his residual Human Qi (Gui Qi or Ghost Qi, 鬼氣) is weak compared to a living person's. Therefore, the Ghost Qi is Yin as it dissipates, while the living person's Qi is Yang. When discussing Qi within the body, in the Lung Channel for example, the reference point is the normal, healthy status of the Qi there. If the Qi is stronger than it is in the normal state, it is Yang, and, naturally, if it is weaker than this, it is Yin. There are twelve parts of the human body that are considered organs in Chinese medicine, six of them are Yin and six are Yang. The Yin organs are the Heart, Lungs, Kidneys, Liver, Spleen, and Pericardium, and the Yang organs are Large Intestine, Small Intestine, Stomach, Gall Bladder, Urinary Bladder, and Triple Burner. Generally speaking, the Qi level of the Yin organs is lower than that of the Yang organs. The Yin organs store Original Essence and process the Essence obtained from food and air, while the Yang organs handle digestion and excretion.

When the Qi in any of your organs is not in its normal state, you feel uncomfortable. If it deviates very much off from the normal state, the organ starts to malfunction and you may become sick. When this happens, the Qi in your entire body is also be affected and you will feel too Yang, perhaps feverish, or too Yin, such as the weakness after diarrhea.

Your body's Qi level is also affected by your natural environment, such as the weather, climate, and seasonal changes. Therefore, when the body's Qi level is classified, the reference point is the level that feels most comfortable for those particular circumstances. Naturally, each of us is a little bit different, and what feels best and most natural for one person may be a bit different from what is right for another person. That is why the doctor will usually ask "how do you feel?" It is according to your own standard that you are judged.

Breathing is closely related to the state of your Qi, and is therefore also considered Yin or Yang. When you exhale you expel air from your lungs, your mind moves outward, and the Qi around the body expands. In the Chinese martial arts, the exhale is generally used to expand the Qi to energize the muscles during an attack. Therefore, you can see that the exhale is Yang—it is expanding, aggressive, and strong. Likewise, based on the same theory, the inhale is considered Yin.

Your breathing is closely related to your emotions. When you lose your temper, your breathing is short and fast, i.e., Yang. When you are sad, your body is more Yin, and you inhale more than you exhale in order to absorb Qi from the air to balance the body's Yin and bring the body back into balance. When you are excited and happy your body is

Yang, and your exhale is longer than your inhale to get rid of the excess Yang that is caused by the excitement.

As mentioned previously, your mind is also closely related to your Qi. Therefore, when your Qi is Yang, your mind is usually also Yang (excited) and vice versa. The mind can also be classified according to the Qi that generated it. The mind (Yi, 意) that is generated from the calm and peaceful Qi obtained from the Original Essence is considered Yin. The mind (Xin, 心) which originates with the food and air essence is emotional, scattered, and excited, and it is considered Yang. The spirit, that is related to the Qi, can also be classified as Yang or Yin based on its origin.

Do not confuse Yin Qi and Yang Qi with Fire Qi (Huo Qi, 火氣) and Water Qi (Shui Qi, 水氣). The Yin and Yang of Qi refers to the level of Qi according to some reference point. However, Water and Fire Qi refers to the quality of the Qi. If you are interested in reading more about the Yin and Yang of Qi, please refer to the Book: *The Root of Chinese Qigong* and *Qigong—The Secret of Youth,* by this author.

The terms Kan (坎) and Li (離) occur frequently in Qigong documents. In the Eight Trigrams, Kan represents "Water" while Li represents "Fire." However, the everyday terms for water and fire are also often used. Kan and Li training has long been of major importance to Qigong practitioners. In order to understand why, you must understand these two words, and the theory behind them.

First you should understand that though Kan-Li and Yin-Yang are related, Kan and Li are not Yin and Yang. Kan is Water, which is able to cool your body down and make it more Yin, while Li is Fire, which warms your body and makes it more Yang. Kan and Li are the methods or causes, while Yin and Yang are the results. When Kan and Li are adjusted and regulated correctly, Yin and Yang will be balanced and interact harmoniously.

Qigong practitioners believe that your body is always too Yang, unless you are sick or have not eaten for a long time, in which case your body may be more Yin. Since your body is always Yang, it is degenerating and burning out. It is believed that this is the cause of aging. If you can use Water to cool down your body, you will be able to slow down the degeneration process and thereby lengthen your life. This is the main reason why Chinese Qigong practitioners have been studying ways to improve the quality of the Water in their bodies, and of reducing the quantity of the Fire. I believe that as a Qigong practitioner you should always keep this subject at the top of your list for study and research. If you earnestly ponder and experiment, you will be able to grasp the knack of adjusting them.

If you want to learn how to adjust them, you must understand that Water and Fire take on many aspects in your body. As mentioned earlier, Qi is classified as Fire and Water. When your Qi is not pure and causes your physical body to heat up and your mental/spiritual body to become unstable (Yang), it is classified as Fire Qi. The Qi that is pure and is able to cool both your physical and spiritual bodies (make them more Yin) is considered Water Qi. However, your body can never be purely Water. Water can cool down the Fire, but it must never totally quench it, because then you would be dead. It is also said that Fire Qi is able to agitate and stimulate the emotions, and from these emotions generate a "mind." This mind is called Xin (心), and is considered the Fire mind, Yang mind, or emotional mind. On the other hand, the mind that Water Qi generates is calm, steady, and wise. This mind is called Yi (意), and is considered to be the Water mind or wisdom mind. If your spirit is nourished by the Fire Qi, although your spirit may be high, it will be scattered and confused (a Yang spirit). Naturally, if the spirit is nourished and raised up by Water Qi, it will be firm and steady (a Yin mind). When your Yi is able to govern your emotional Xin effectively, your will (strong emotional intention) can be firm.

You can see from this discussion that your Qi is the main cause of the Yin and Yang state of your physical body, your mind, and your spirit. To regulate your body's Yin and Yang, you must learn how to regulate your body's Water and Fire Qi, but in order to do this efficiently you must know their sources.

Once you have grasped the concepts of Yin-Yang and Kan-Li, then you have to think about how to adjust Kan and Li so that you can balance the Yin and Yang in your body.

Theoretically, a Qigong practitioner would like to keep his body in a state of Yin-Yang balance, which means the "center" point of the Yin and Yang forces. This center point is commonly called "Wuji" (無極) (no extremities). It is believed that Wuji is the original, natural state where Yin and Yang are not differentiated. In the Wuji state, nature is peaceful and calm. In the Wuji state, all of the Yin and Yang forces have gradually combined harmoniously and disappeared. When this Wuji theory is applied to human beings, it is the final goal of Qigong practice where your mind is neutral and absolutely calm. The Wuji state makes it possible for you to find the origin of your life, and to combine your Qi with the Qi of nature.

The ultimate goal and purpose of Qigong practice is to find this peaceful and natural state. In order to reach this goal, you must first understand your body's Yin and Yang so that you can balance them by adjusting your Kan and Li. Only when your Yin and Yang are balanced will you be able to find the center balance point, the Wuji state.

Theoretically, between the two extremes of Yin and Yang are millions of paths (i.e., different Kan and Li methods) that can lead you to the neutral center. This accounts for the hundreds of different styles of Qigong which have been created over the years. You can see that the theory of Yin and Yang and the methods of Kan and Li are the root of training all Chinese Qigong styles. Without this root, the essence of Qigong practice would be lost.

Three Treasures—Jing, Qi, and Shen 三寶 - 精、氣、神

Before you start any Qigong training you must also understand the three treasures of your body (San Bao, 三寶): Jing (精) (Essence), Qi (氣) (Internal Energy), and Shen (神) (Spirit). They are also called the three origins or the three roots (San Yuan, 三元),

because they are considered the origins and roots of your life. Jing means Essence, the most original and refined part. Jing is the original source and most basic part of every living thing, and determines its nature and characteristics. It is the root of life. Sperm is called Jing Zi (精子), which means "Essence of the Son," because it contains the Jing of the father that is passed on to his son (or daughter) and becomes the son's Jing.

Qi, known as bioelectricity today, is the internal energy of your body. It is like the electricity that passes through a machine to keep it running. Qi comes either from the conversion of the Jing that you have received from your parents, or from the food you eat and the air you breathe.

Shen is the center of your mind and being. It is what makes you human, because animals do not have a Shen. The Shen in your body must be nourished by your Qi or energy. When your Qi is full, your Shen will be enlivened.

Chinese meditators and Qigong practitioners believe that the body contains two general types of Qi. The first type is called Pre-Birth Qi or Pre-Heaven Qi (Xian Tian Qi, 先天氣), and it comes from converted Original Jing (Yuan Jing, 元精), which you get from your parents at conception. The second type, called Post-Birth Qi or Post Heaven Qi (Hou Tian Qi, 後天氣), is drawn from the Jing of the food and air we take in. When this Qi flows or is led to the brain, it can energize the Shen and soul. This energized and raised Shen is able to govern and lead the Qi throughout the entire body.

Each one of these three elements or treasures has its own root. You must know the roots so that you can strengthen and protect your three treasures.

1. Your body requires many kinds of Jing. Except for the Jing which you inherit from your parents, called Original Jing (Yuan Jing, 元精), all other Jings must be obtained from food and air. Among all of these Jings, Original Jing is the most important one. It is the root and the seed of your life, and your basic strength. If your parents were strong and healthy, your Original Jing will be strong and healthy, you will have a strong foundation on which to grow. The Chinese people believe that in order to stay healthy and live a long life, you must protect and maintain this Jing.

   According to Chinese medicine, the root of Original Jing before your birth was in your parents. After birth, this Original Jing stays in its residence—the kidneys, which are considered the root of your Jing. When you keep this root strong, you will have sufficient Original Jing to supply to your body. Although you cannot increase the amount of Original Jing you have, Qigong training can improve the quality of your Jing. Qigong can also teach you how to convert your Jing into Original Qi more efficiently, and how to use this Qi effectively.

   If we analyze the concept of Jing from a modern physical scientific point of view, we might postulate that Jing is in the genetic material that we inherited from our parents. From this material, the structure and health of one person differs from all others. The different genes controls the different levels of hormones in different people. When Chinese medicine says that the Original Jing is stored in the kidneys, it implies the hormones which are produced in the adrenal glands. According to Chinese medicine, there is no record of the endocrine glands. This implies that Chinese medicine has never understood the function of the endocrine. In my opinion, the Jing (essence) is stored in all of the endocrine glands. I believe that the most significant gland that stores the essence and affects the level of the entire body's Jing (hormone production) is the pituitary gland (corresponding to the Upper Dan Tian).

2. According to Chinese medicine and Qigong, Qi is converted both from the Jing that you have inherited from your parents and from the Jing that you draw from the food and air you breathe. Qi that is converted from the Original Jing which you inherited is called Original Qi (Yuan Qi, 元氣).[14] Just as Original Jing is the most important type of Jing, Original Qi is the most important type of Qi. It is pure and of high quality, while the Qi from food and air may make your body too positive or too negative, depending on how and where you absorb it. When you retain and protect your Original Jing, you will be able to generate Original Qi in a pure, continuous stream. As a Qigong practitioner, you must know how to convert your Original Jing into Original Qi in a smooth, steady stream.

Since your Original Qi comes from your Original Jing, they both have the kidneys for their root. When your kidneys are strong, the Original Jing is strong, and the Original Qi converted from this Original Jing will also be full and strong. This Qi resides in the Lower Dan Tian in your abdomen. Once you learn how to convert your Original Jing, you will be able to supply your body with all the Qi it needs.

Again, if we analyze the above concepts, we can see that the Essence here means the hormone level that is produced from the adrenal glands on the top of your kidneys. In fact, we have already seen that I consider the pituitary gland to be considered the master of the glands, and when the hormone production in this gland is high, the hormone production of all other endocrine glands will also be high. When the hormone level of the body is high, the Qi is abundant and the circulation is smooth. When the hormone production level is high in the pituitary gland, the spirit (Shen, 神) residing in the center of your brain will be high. When the spirit is high, it is able to strongly and smoothly direct the Qi circulating in the body for functioning, repair and healing. This results in the development of spiritual healing science.

3. Shen (i.e. spirit, 神) is the force that keeps you alive. It has no substance, but it gives expression and appearance to your Jing. Shen is also the control tower

for the Qi. When your Shen is strong, your Qi is strong and you can lead it efficiently. The root of Shen (Spirit) is your mind (Yi, or intention). When your brain is energized and stimulated, your mind will be more aware and you will be able to concentrate more intensely. Also, your Shen will be raised. Advanced Qigong practitioners believe that your brain must always be sufficiently nourished by your Qi. It is the Qi that keeps your mind clear and concentrated. With an abundant Qi supply, the mind can be energized, and can raise the Shen and enhance your vitality.

The deeper levels of Qigong training include the conversion of Jing into Qi (Lian Jing Hua Qi, 練精化氣), which is then led to the brain to raise the Shen (Lian Qi Hua Shen, 練氣化神). This process is called "Huan Jing Bu Nao" (還精補腦) and means "return the Jing to nourish the brain." When Qi is led to the head, it stays at the Upper Dan Tian (at the center of the forehead), which is the residence of your Shen. Qi and Shen are mutually related. When your Shen is weak, your Qi is weak, and your body will deteriorate rapidly. Shen is the headquarters of Qi. Likewise, Qi supports the Shen, energizing it and keeping it sharp, clear, and strong. If the Qi in your body is weak, your Shen will also be weak.

From the viewpoint of science, in order to maintain a high hormone production level, you must continue to supply bioelectricity to the pituitary gland. Without this basic energy, the gland will not function adequately. Therefore, one of the main Qigong practices is learning, through meditation, how to lead the Qi to the brain and nourish the pituitary gland.

From the above discussion, you can see that in order to have a healthy and strong body, you must first learn how to maintain the Yin and Yang balance in your body. In addition, you should also learn how to adjust or regulate your body, allowing you to harmonize it with the natural environment. Furthermore, you should learn how to retain and generate your Jing, strengthen and smooth your Qi flow, and enlighten your Shen. That means you should learn how to maintain the hormone production of your body, how to store the Qi in your Lower Dan Tian (battery) and smoothly circulate it in your body, and how to lead the Qi to the brain to nourish your Spirit. If you are interested in the further pursuit of enlightenment, then you must learn how to regulate your mind to a neutral state and build up a Spiritual Embryo (Sheng Tai, 聖胎). From the cultivation of this Spiritual Embryo, you will be able to separate your spiritual body and your physical body. If you are interested in this subject, please refer to *Qigong—The Secret of Youth*, by this author.

Qigong Training Theory 氣功訓練理論

Every Qigong form or practice has its special training purpose and theory. If you do not know the purpose and theory, you have lost the root (meaning) of the practice.

Therefore, as a Qigong practitioner, you must continue to ponder and practice until you understand the root of every set or form.

Remember that getting the gold is not enough. Like the boy in the old Chinese story, you should concern yourself with learning the knack of turning the rock into gold. You can see that getting the gold is simply gaining the flowers and branches, and there can be no growth. However, if you have the knack which is the theory, then you will have the root, and you may continue to grow by yourself.

Now that you have learned the basic theory of the Qigong practice, let us discuss the general training principles. In Chinese Qigong society, it is commonly known that in order to reach the goal of Qigong practice, you must learn how to regulate the body (Tiao Shen, 調身), regulate the breathing (Tiao Xi, 調息), regulate the emotional mind (Tiao Xin, 調心), regulate the Qi (Tiao Qi, 調氣), and regulate the spirit (Tiao Shen, 調神). Tiao in Chinese is constructed from two words, "言" (Yan, means speaking or talking) and "周" (Zhou, means round or complete). That means the roundness (i.e. harmony) or the completeness is accomplished by negotiation. Like an out-of-tune in piano, you must adjust it and make it harmonize with others. This implies that, when you are regulating one of the above five processes, you must also coordinate and harmonize the other four regulating elements.

Regulating the body includes understanding how to find and build the root of the body, as well as the root of the individual forms you are practicing. To build a firm root, you must know how to keep your center, how to balance your body, and most important of all, how to relax so that the Qi can flow.

To regulate your breathing, you must learn how to breathe so that your respiration and your mind mutually correspond and cooperate. When you breathe this way, your mind will be able to attain peace more quickly, and therefore concentrate more easily on leading the Qi.

Regulating the mind involves learning how to keep your mind calm, peaceful, and centered, so that you can judge situations objectively and lead Qi to the desired places. The mind is the main key to success in Qigong practice.

Regulating the Qi is one of the ultimate goals of Qigong practice. In order to regulate your Qi effectively, you must first have regulated your body breathing, and mind. Only then will your mind be clear enough to sense how the Qi is distributed in your body, and understand how to adjust it.

For Buddhist and Daoist priests, who seek enlightenment or Buddhahood regulating the spirit (Shen) is the final goal of Qigong. This enables them to maintain a neutral, objective perspective of life, and this perspective is the eternal life of the Buddha. The average Qigong practitioner has lesser goals. He raises his spirit in order to increase his concentration and enhance his vitality. This makes it possible for him to lead Qi effectively throughout his entire body so that it carries out the managing and guarding duties. This maintains health and slows the aging process.

If you understand these few things, you will be able to quickly enter into the field of Qigong. Without all of these important elements, your training will be ineffective and your time will be wasted.

Before you start training, you must first understand that all of the training originates in your mind. You must have a clear idea of what you are doing, and your mind must be calm, centered, and balanced. This also implies that your feeling, sensing, and judgment must be objective and accurate. This requires emotional balance and a clear mind. This takes a lot of hard work, but once you have reached this level you will have built the root of your physical training, and your Yi (mind) will be able to lead your Qi throughout your physical body.

1. Regulating the Body (Tiao Shen, 調身)

When you learn any Qigong, either moving or still, the first step is to learn the correct postures or movements. After you have learned the postures and movements, you learn how to improve them until you can perform the forms accurately. Then, you start to regulate your body until it has reached the stage that can provide the best environment for the Qi to build up or to circulate.

In Still Qigong practice or Soft Qigong movement, this means to adjust your body until it is in the most comfortable and relaxed state. This implies that your body must be centered and balanced. If it is not, you will be tense and uneasy, and this will affect the judgment of your Yi and the circulation of your Qi. In Chinese medical society, it is said: "(When) shape (body's posture) is not correct, then the Qi will not be smooth. (When) the Qi is not smooth, the Yi (wisdom mind) will not be peaceful. (When) the Yi is not peaceful, then the Qi is disordered."[15] You should understand that the relaxation of your body originates with your Yi. Therefore, before you can relax your body, you must first relax or regulate your mind (Yi). This is called "Shen Xin Ping Heng" (身心平衡), which means "Body and heart (i.e., mind) balanced." The body and the mind are mutually related. A relaxed and balanced body helps your Yi to relax and concentrate. When your Yi is at peace and can judge things accurately, your body will be relaxed, balanced, centered, and rooted. Only when you are rooted, then you will be able to raise up your spirit of vitality.

Relaxation 放鬆

Relaxation is one of the major keys to success in Qigong. You should remember that only when you are relaxed will all your Qi channels be open. In order to be relaxed, your Yi must first be relaxed and calm. When the Yi coordinates with your breathing, your body will be able to relax.

In Qigong practice, there are three levels of relaxation. The first level is the external physical relaxation, or postural relaxation. This is a very superficial level and almost anyone can reach it. It consists of adopting a comfortable stance and avoiding unnecessary strain in how you stand and move. The second level is the relaxation of the muscles and tendons. To do this your Yi must be directed deep into the muscles and tendons. This relaxation will help open your Qi channels, and will allow the Qi to sink and accumulate in the Dan Tian.

The final stage is the relaxation that reaches the internal organs and the bone marrow. Remember, only if you can relax deep into your body, will your mind be able to lead the Qi there. Only at this stage will the Qi be able to reach everywhere in the body. Then you will feel transparent—as if your whole body had disappeared. If you can reach this level of relaxation, you will be able to communicate with your organs and use Qigong to adjust or regulate the Qi disorders which are giving you problems. You will also be able to protect your organs more effectively, and therefore slow down their deterioration.

Rooting 紮根

In all Qigong practice it is very important to be rooted. Being rooted means to be stable and in firm contact with the ground. If you want to push a car, you must be rooted so the force you exert into the car will be balanced by an opposing force into the ground. If you are not rooted, when you push the car you will only push yourself away, and not move the car. Your root is made up of your body's root, center, and balance.

Before you can develop your root, you must first relax and let your body "settle." As you relax, the tension in the various parts of your body will dissolve, and you will find a comfortable way to stand. You will stop fighting the ground to keep your body up, and will learn to rely on your body's structure to support itself. This lets the muscles relax even more. Since your body isn't struggling to stand up, your Yi won't be pushing upward, and your body, mind, and Qi will all be able to sink. If you let dirty water sit quietly, the impurities will gradually settle down to the bottom, leaving the water above it clear. In the same way, if you relax your body enough to let it settle, your Qi will sink to your Dan Tian, and the Bubbling Wells (Yongquan, K-1, 湧泉) in your feet and your mind will become clear. Then you can begin to develop your root.

To root your body you must imitate a tree and grow an invisible root under your feet. This will give you a firm root to keep you stable in your training. Your root must be wide as well as deep. Naturally, your Yi must grow first, because it is the Yi which leads the Qi. Your Yi must be able to lead the Qi to your feet, and be able to communicate with the ground. Only when your Yi can communicate with the ground will your Qi be able to grow beyond your feet and enter the ground to build the root. The Bubbling Well cavity is the gate that enables your Qi to communicate with the ground.

After you have gained your root, you must learn how to keep your center. A stable center will make your Qi develop evenly and uniformly. If you lost this center, your Qi will not be evenly led. In order to keep your body centered, you must first center your Yi, and then align your body with it. Only under these conditions will the Qigong forms you practice have their root. Your mental and physical centers are the keys that enable you to lead your Qi beyond your body.

Balance is the product of rooting and centering. Balance includes balancing the Qi and the physical body. It does not matter which aspect of balance you are dealing with, first you must balance your Yi, and only then can you balance your Qi and your physical body. If your Yi is balanced, it can help you to make accurate judgments, and therefore to correct the path of the Qi flow.

Rooting includes not just rooting the body, but also the form or movement. The root of any form or movement is found in its purpose or principle. For example, in certain Qigong exercises you want to lead the Qi to your palms. In order to do this, you may imagine that you are pushing an object forward while keeping your muscles relaxed. In this exercise, your elbows must be down to build the sense of root for the push. If you raise the elbows, you lose the sense of "intention" of the movement, because the push would be ineffective if you were pushing something for real. Since the intention or purpose of the movement is its reason for being, you now have a scattered, purposeless movement, and you have no reason to lead Qi in any particular way. Therefore, in this case, the elbow is the root of the movement.

2. Regulating the Breath (Tiao Xi, 調息)

Regulating the breath means to regulate your breathing until it is calm, smooth, and peaceful. Only when you have reached this point will you be able to make the breathing deep, slender, long, and soft, which is required for successful Qigong practice.

Breathing is affected by your emotions. For example, when you are angry or excited, you exhale more strongly than you inhale. When you are sad, you inhale more strongly than you exhale. When your mind is peaceful and calm, your inhalation and exhalation are relatively equal. In order to keep your breathing calm, peaceful, and steady, your mind and emotions must first be calm and neutral. Therefore, in order to regulate your breathing, you must first regulate your mind.

The other side of the coin is that you can use your breathing to control your Yi. When your breathing is uniform, it is as if you were hypnotizing your Yi, which helps to calm it. You can see that Yi and breathing are interdependent, and that they cooperate with each other. Deep and calm breathing relaxes you and keeps your mind clear. It fills your lungs with plenty of air, so that your brain and entire body have an adequate supply of oxygen. In addition, deep and complete breathing lets the diaphragm to move up and down, which massages and stimulates the internal organs. For this reason, deep breathing exercises are also called "internal organ exercises."

Deep and complete breathing does not mean that you inhale and exhale to the maximum. This would cause the lungs and the surrounding muscles to tense up, which in turn would keep the air from circulating freely, and hinder the absorption of oxygen. Without enough oxygen, your mind becomes scattered, and the rest of your body tenses up. In correct breathing, you inhale and exhale to about 70% or 80% of capacity, so that your lungs stay relaxed.

You can conduct an easy experiment. Inhale deeply so that your lungs are completely full, and time how long you can hold your breath. Then try inhaling to only about 70% of your capacity, and see how long you can hold your breath. You will find that with the latter method you can last much longer than the first one. This is simply because the lungs and the surrounding muscles are relaxed. When they are relaxed, the rest of your body and your mind can also relax, which significantly decreases your need for oxygen. Therefore, when you regulate your breathing, the first priority is to keep your lungs relaxed and calm.

When training, your mind must first be calm so that your breathing can be regulated. When the breathing is regulated, your mind is able to reach a higher level of calmness. This calmness can again help you to regulate the breathing, until your mind is deep. After you have trained for a long time, your breathing will be full and slender, and your mind will be very clear. It is said: "Xin Xi Xiang Yi" (心息相依), which means "Heart (Mind) and breathing (are) interdependent." When you reach this meditative state, your heartbeat slows down, and your mind is very clear; you have entered the sphere of real meditation.

An ancient Daoist named Li, Qing-An (李清庵) said: "Regulating breathing means to regulate the real breathing until (you) stop."[16] This means that regulating correctly means regulating is no longer necessary. Real regulating is no longer a conscious process, but has become so natural that it can be accomplished without conscious effort. In other words, although you start by consciously regulating your breath, you must reach the point where the regulating happens naturally, and you no longer need to think about it. When you breathe, if you concentrate your mind on your breathing, then it is not true regulating, because the Qi in your lungs will become stagnant. When you reach the level of true regulating, you don't have to pay attention to it, and you can use your mind efficiently to lead the Qi. Remember, wherever the Yi is, there is the Qi. If the Yi stops in one spot, the Qi will be stagnant. It is the Yi which leads the Qi and makes it move. Therefore, when you are in a state of correct breath regulation, your mind is free. There is no sound stagnation, urgency, or hesitation, and you can finally be calm and peaceful.

You can see that when the breath is regulated correctly, the Qi will also be regulated. They are mutually related and cannot be separated. This idea is explained frequently in the Daoist literature. The Daoist Guang Cheng Zi (廣成子) said: "One exhale, the Earth Qi rises; one inhale, the Heaven Qi descends; real man's (meaning one who has attained the real Dao) repeated breathing at the navel, then my real Qi is naturally connected."[17] This says that when you breathe, you should move your abdomen, as if you were breathing from your navel. The earth Qi is the negative (Yin) energy from your kidneys, and the sky Qi is the positive (Yang) energy that comes from the food you eat and the air you breathe. When you breathe from the navel, these two Qi's will connect and combine. Some people think that they know what Qi is, but they really don't. Once you connect the two Qi's, you will know what the "real" Qi is, and you may become a "real" man, which means to attain the Dao.

The Daoist book *Chang Dao Zhen Yan* (唱道真言) (*Song (of the) Dao (with) Real Words*) says: "One exhale one inhale to communicate Qi's function, one movement one calmness is the same as (i.e., is the source of) creation and variation."[18] The first part of this statement again implies that the functioning of Qi is connected with the breathing. The second part of this sentence means that all creation and variation come from the interaction of movement (Yang) and calmness (Yin). *Huang Ting Jing* (黃庭經) (*Yellow Yard Classic*) says: "Breathe Original Qi to seek immortality."[19] In China, the traditional Daoists wore yellow robes, and they meditated in a "yard" or hall. This sentence means that in order to reach the goal of immortality, you must seek to find and understand the Original Qi which comes from the Dan Tian through correct breathing.

Moreover, the Daoist Wu Zhen Ren (伍真人) said: "Use the Post-Birth breathing to look for the real person's (i.e., the immortal's) breathing place."[20] In this sentence, it is clear that in order to locate the immortal breathing place (the Dan Tian), on which you must rely and know how to regulate your Post-Birth, or natural breathing. Through regulating your Post-Birth breathing, you will gradually be able to locate the residence of the Qi (the Dan Tian), and eventually you will be able to use your Dan Tian to breath like the immortal Daoists. Finally, in the Daoist song *Ling Yuan Da Dao Ge* (靈源大道歌) (*The Great Daoist Song of the Spirit's Origin*) it is said: "The Originals (Original Jing, Qi, and Shen) are internally transported peacefully, so that you can become real (immortal); (if you) depend (only) on external breathing (you) will not reach the end (goal)."[21] From this song, you can see the internal breathing (breathing at the Dan Tian) is the key to training your three treasures and finally reaching immortality. However, you must first know how to regulate your external breathing correctly.

All of these songs emphasize the importance of breathing. There are eight key words for air breathing that a Qigong practitioner should follow during his practice. Once you understand them, you will be able to substantially shorten the time needed to reach your Qigong goals. These eight key words are: 1. Calm (Jing, 靜); 2. Slender (Xi, 細); 3. Deep (Shen, 深); 4. Long (Chang, 長); 5. Continuous (You, 悠); 6. Uniform (Yun, 勻); 7. Slow (Huan, 緩), and 8. Soft (Mian, 綿). These key words are self-explanatory, and with a little thought you should be able to understand them.

3. Regulating the Mind (Tiao Xin, 調心)

It is said in Daoist society that: "(When) large Dao is taught, first stop thought; when thought is not stopped, (the lessons are) in vain."[22] This means that when you first practice Qigong, the most difficult training is to stop your thinking. The final goal for your mind is "the thought of no thought" (Wu Nian Zhi Nian, 無念之念). Your mind does not think of the past, present, or future. Your mind is completely separated from influences of the present such as worry, happiness, and sadness. Then your mind can be calm and steady, and can finally gain peace. Only when you are in the state of "the thought of no thought" will you be relaxed and able to sense calmly and accurately.

Regulating your mind means using your consciousness to stop the activity in your mind in order to set it free from the bondage of ideas, emotion, and conscious thought. When you reach this level your mind will be calm, peaceful, empty, and light. Then your mind has actually reached the goal of relaxation. Only when you reach this stage will you be able to relax deep into your marrow and internal organs. Only then will your mind be clear enough to see (feel) the internal Qi circulation and to communicate with your Qi and organs. In Daoist society, this state is called, "Nei Shi Gongfu" (內視功夫), which means the Gongfu of internal vision.

When you reach this real relaxation, you may be able to sense the different elements that make up your body: solid matter, liquids, gases, energy, and spirit. You may even be able to see or feel the different colors that are associated with your five organs: green (liver), white (lungs), black (kidneys), yellow (spleen), and red (heart).

Once your mind is relaxed and regulated and you can sense your internal organs, you may decide to study the Five Element theory. This is a very profound subject, and it is sometimes interpreted differently by Oriental physicians and Qigong practitioners. When understood properly, the theory can give you a method of analyzing the interrelationships between your organs and help you devise ways to correct imbalances.

For example, the lungs correspond to the element Metal, and the heart to the element Fire. Metal (the lungs) can be used to adjust the heat of the Fire (the heart), because metal can take a large quantity of heat away from fire, (and thus cool down the heart). When you feel uneasy or have heartburn (excess fire in the heart), you may use deep breathing to calm the uneasy emotions down or cool off the heartburn.

Naturally, it will take much practice to reach this level. In the beginning, you should not have any ideas or intentions, because they will make it harder for your mind to relax and empty itself of thoughts. Once you are in a state of "no thought," place your attention on your Lower Dan Tian (Xia Dan Tian, 下丹田). It is said "Yi Shou Dan Tian" (意守丹田), which means "The Mind is kept on the Dan Tian." The Dan Tian is the origin and residence of your Qi. Your mind can build up the Qi here (start the fire, Qi Huo, 起火), then lead the Qi anywhere you wish, and finally lead the Qi back to its residence. When your mind is on the Dan Tian, your Qi will always have a root. When you keep this root, your Qi will be strong and full, and it will go where you want it to go. You can see that when you practice Qigong, your mind cannot be completely empty and relaxed. If you can find the firmness within the relaxation, then you can reach your goal.

In Qigong training, it is said: "Use your Yi (Mind) to lead your Qi" (Yi Yi Yin Qi) (以意引氣). Notice the word "lead". Qi behaves like water—it cannot be pushed, but it can be led. When Qi is led, it will flow smoothly and without stagnation. When it is pushed, it will flood and enter the wrong paths. Remember wherever your Yi goes first, the Qi will naturally follow. For example, if you intend to lift an object, this intention is your Yi. This Yi will lead the Qi to the arms to energize the physical muscles, and then the object can be lifted.

It is said: "Your Yi cannot be on your Qi. Once your Yi is on your Qi, the Qi is stagnant."[23] When you want to walk from one spot to another, you must first mobilize your intention and direct it to the goal, then your body will follow. The mind must always be ahead of the body. If your mind stays on your body, you will not be able to move.

In Qigong training, the first thing is to know what Qi is. If you do not know what Qi is, how will you be able to lead it? Once you know what Qi is and experience it, then your Yi will have something to lead. The next thing in Qigong training is knowing how your Yi communicates with your Qi. That means that your Yi should be able to sense and feel the Qi flow and understand how strong and smooth it is. In Taiji Qigong society, it is commonly said that your Yi must "listen" to your Qi and "understand" it. Listen means to pay careful attention to what you sense and feel. The more you pay attention, the better you will be able to understand. Only after you understand the Qi pattern will your Yi be able to set up the strategy. In Qigong your mind or Yi must generate the idea (visualize your intention), which is like an order to your Qi to complete a certain mission.

The more your Yi communicates with your Qi, the more efficiently the Qi can be led. For this reason, as a Qigong beginner you must first learn about Yi and Qi, and also learn how to help them communicate effectively. Yi is the key in Qigong practice. Without this Yi you would not be able to lead your Qi, let alone build up the strength of the Qi or circulate it throughout your entire body.

Remember when the Yi is strong, the Qi is strong, and when the Yi is weak, the Qi is weak. Therefore, the first step in Qigong training is to develop your Yi. The first secret of a strong Yi is calmness. When you are calm, you can see things clearly and not be disturbed by surrounding distractions. With your mind calm, you will be able to concentrate.

Confucius (Kong Zi, 孔子) said: "First you must be calm, then your mind can be steady. Once your mind is steady, then you are at peace. Only when you are at peace are you able to think and finally gain."[24] This process is also applied in meditation or Qigong exercise: First Calm, then Steady, Peace, Think, and finally Gain. When you practice Qigong, first you must learn to be emotionally calm. Once calm, you will be able to see what you want and firm your mind (steady). This firm and steady mind is your intention or Yi (it is how your Yi is generated). Only after you know what you really want will your mind gain peace and be able to relax emotionally and physically. Once you have reached this step, you must then concentrate or think in order to execute your intention. Under this thoughtful and concentrated mind, your Qi will follow and you will be able to gain what you wish.

However, the most difficult part of regulating the mind is learning how to neutralize the thoughts that keep coming back to bother you. This is especially true in still meditation practice. In still meditation, once you have entered a deep, profound meditative state, new thoughts, fantasies, your imagination, or any guilt from what you have done in the past that is hidden behind your mask will emerge and bother you. Normally, the first step of the regulating process is to stop new fantasies and images. Then, you must deal with your conscious mind. That means you must learn how to remove the mask from your face. Only then will you see yourself clearly. Therefore, the first step is to know yourself. Next, you must learn how to handle the problem instead of continuing to avoid it.

There are many ways of regulating your mind. However, the most important key to success is to use your wisdom mind to analyze the situation and find the solution. Do not let your emotional mind govern your thinking. Here, I would like to share with you a few stories about regulating the mind. Hopefully these stories can provide you with a guideline for your own regulation.

In China many centuries ago, two monks were walking side by side down a muddy road when they came upon a large puddle that completely blocked the road. A very beautiful lady in a lovely gown stood at the edge of the puddle, unable to go further without spoiling her clothes.

Without hesitation, one of the monks picked her up and carried her across the puddle, set her down on the other side, and continued on his way. Many hours later when the two monks were preparing to camp for the night, the second monk turned to the first and said, "I can no longer hold this back, I'm quite angry at you! We are not supposed to look at women, particularly pretty ones, never mind touch them. Why did you do that?" The first monk replied, "Brother, I left the woman at the mud puddle; why are you still carrying her?"

From this story, you can see that often, the thought that bothers you is created by nobody but yourself. If you can use your wisdom mind to govern yourself, many times you can set your mind free from emotional bondage regardless of the situation.

It is true that frequently the mind bothers or enslaves you to the desire for material enjoyment or money. From this desire, you misunderstand the meaning of life. A really happy life comes from satisfaction of both material and spiritual needs.

Have you ever thought about what the real meaning of your life is? What is the real goal for your life? Are you enslaved by money, power, or love? What will make you truly happy?

I remember a story one of my professors at Taiwan University told me: "There was a jail with a prisoner in it," he said, "who was surrounded by mountains of money. He kept counting the money and feeling so happy about his life, thinking that he was the richest man in the whole world. A man passing by saw him and said through the tiny window: 'Why are you so happy, you are in prison?' Do you know that? The prisoner laughed: "No! No! It is not that I am inside the jail, it is that you are outside of the jail!"

How do you feel about this story? Do you want to be a prisoner and a slave to money, or do you want to be the real you and feel free internally? Think and be happy.

There is another story which was told to me by one of my students. Ever since I heard this story, it has always offered me a new guideline for my life. This new guideline is to appreciate what you have; only then will you have a peaceful mind. This does not mean you should not be aggressive in pursuing a better life. Keep pursuing by creating a new target and a new path for your life. It is Yang. However, often you will be depressed and discouraged from obstacles on this path. Therefore, you must also learn how to comfort yourself and appreciate what you already have. This is Yin. Only if you have both Yin and Yang can your life be happy and meaningful.

Long ago, there was a servant who served a bad tempered and impatient master. It did not matter how he tried, he was always blamed and beaten by this master. However, it was the strange truth that the servant was always happy, and his master was always sad and depressed.

One day, there was a kind man who could not understand this phenomena, and finally decided to ask this servant why he was always happy even though he was treated so badly. The servant replied: "Everyone has one day of life each day; half of the day is spent awake and the other half is spent sleeping. Although in the daytime, I am a servant and my master treats me badly, in the nighttime, I always dream that I am a king and there are thousands of servants serving me luxuriously. Look at my master: In the daytime, he is mad, depressed, greedy, and unhappy. In the nighttime, he has nightmares and cannot even have one night of nice rest. I really feel sorry for my master. Comparing me to him, I am surely happier than he is."

Friends, what do you think about this story? You are the only one responsible for your happiness. If you are not satisfied, and always complain about what you have obtained, you will be on the course of forever-unhappiness. It is said in Western society: "If you smile, the whole world smiles with you, but if you cry, you cry alone." What a true saying!

4. Regulating the Qi (Tiao Qi, 調氣)

Before you can regulate your Qi, you must first regulate your body, breath, and mind. If you compare your body to a battlefield, then your mind is like the general who generates ideas and controls the situation, and your breathing is the strategy. Your Qi is like the soldiers who are led to the most advantageous places on the battlefield. All four elements are necessary and all four must be coordinated with each other if you are to win the war against sickness and aging.

If you want to arrange your soldiers most effectively for battle, you must know which area of the battlefield is most important, and where you are weakest (where your Qi is deficient) and need to send reinforcements. If you have more soldiers than you need in one area (excessive Qi), then you can send them somewhere else where the ranks are thin. As a general, you must also know how many soldiers are available for the battle, and how many you will need for protecting yourself and your headquarters. To be successful, not only do you need good strategy (breathing), but you also need to communicate and understand the situation effectively with your troops, or all of your strategy will be in vain. When your Yi (the general) knows how to regulate the body (knows the battlefield), how to regulate breathing (set up the strategy), and how to effectively regulate Qi (direct your soldiers), you will be able to reach the final goal of Qigong training.

In order to regulate your Qi so that it moves smoothly in the correct paths, you need more than just efficient Yi-Qi communication. You also need to know how to generate Qi. If you do not have enough Qi in your body, how can you regulate it? In a battle, if you do not have enough soldiers to set up your strategy, you have already lost.

When you practice Qigong, you must first train to make you Qi flow naturally and smoothly. There are some Qigong exercises in which you intentionally hold your Yi, and thus hold your Qi, in a specific area. As a beginner, however, you should first learn not to make a Qi dam but to make the Qi flow smoothly (Qi dams are commonly used in external martial Qigong training).

In order to make Qi flow naturally and smoothly, your Yi must first be relaxed. Only when your Yi is relaxed will your body be relaxed and the Qi channels open for the Qi to circulate. Then you must coordinate your Qi flow with your breathing. Breathing regularly and calmly will make your Yi calm, and allow your body to relax even more.

5. Regulating Spirit (Tiao Shen, 調神)

There is one thing that is more important than anything else in a battle, and that is fighting spirit. You may have the best general, who knows the battlefield well and is also an expert strategist, but if his soldiers do not have a high fighting spirit (morale), he might still lose. Remember, spirit is the center and root of a fight. When you keep this center, one soldier can be equal to ten soldiers. When his spirit is high, a soldier will obey his orders accurately and willingly, and his general will be able to control the situation efficiently. In a battle, in order for a soldier to have this kind of morale, he must know why he is fighting, how to fight, and what he can expect after the fight. Under these conditions, he will know what he is doing and why, and this understanding will raise up his spirit, strengthen his will, and increase his patience and endurance.

Shen, which is the Chinese term for spirit, originates from the Yi (the general). When the Shen is strong, the Yi is firm. When the Yi is firm, the Shen will be steady and calm. The Shen is the mental part of a soldier. When the Shen is high, the Qi is strong and easily directed. When the Qi is strong, the Shen is also strong.

To religious Qigong practitioners, the goal of regulating the spirit is to set the spirit free from the bondage of the physical body, and thus reach the stage of Buddhahood or enlightenment. To layman practitioners, the goal of regulating the spirit is to keep the spirit of living high to prevent the body from getting sick and deteriorating. It is often seen that, before a person retires, he has good health. However, once retired, he will get sick easily and his physical condition will deteriorate quickly. When you are working, your spirit remains high and alert. This keeps the Qi circulating smoothly in the body.

All of these training concepts and procedures are common to all Chinese Qigong. To reach a deep level of understanding and penetrate to the essence of any Qigong practice, you should always keep these five training principles in mind and examine them for deeper levels of meaning. This is the only way to gain the real mental and physical health benefits from your training. Always remember that Qigong training is not just the forms. Your feelings and comprehension are the essential roots of the entire training. This Yin side of the training has no limit, and the deeper you understand, the better you will see how much more there is to know.

1-6. How to Use This Book 讀此書之態度

When you practice any Qigong, you must first ask: What, Why, and How. "What" means: "What am I looking for?" "What do I expect?" and "What should I do?" Then you must ask: "Why do I need it?" "Why does it work?" "Why must I do it this way instead of that way?" Finally, you must determine: "How does it work?" "How much have I advanced toward my goal?" And "How will I be able to advance further?"

It is very important to understand what you are practicing, not just automatically to repeat what you have learned. Understanding is the root of any work. With understanding you will be able to know your goal. Once you know your goal, your mind can be firm and steady. With this understanding, you will be able to see why something has happened, and what the principles and theories behind it are. Without all of this, your work will be done blindly, and it will be a long and painful process. Only when you are sure what your target is and why you need to reach it should you raise the question of how you are going to accomplish it. The answers to all of these questions form the root of your practice, and will help you to avoid the bewilderment and confusion that uncertainty brings. If you keep this root, you will be able to apply the theory and make it grow—you will know how to create. Without this root, what you learn will be only branches and flowers, and in time they will wither.

In China there is a story about an old man who was able to change a piece of rock into gold. One day, a boy came to see him and asked for his help. The old man said: "Boy! What do you want? Gold? I can give you all of the gold you want." The boy replied: "No, Master, what I want is not your gold. What I want is the trick of how to change the rock into gold!" When you just have gold, you can spend it all and become poor again. If you have the knowledge of how to make gold, you will never be poor. For the same reason, when you learn Qigong you should learn the theory and principle behind it, not just the practice. Understanding theory and principle will not only shorten your time of pondering and practice, but also enable you to practice most efficiently.

One of the hardest parts of the training process is learning how actually to do the forms correctly. Every Qigong movement has its special meaning and purpose. In order to make sure your movements or forms are correct, it is best to work with the tape and book together. There are some important aspects which you may not be able to pick up from reading, but once you see them, they will be clear. There are other important ideas for which it was impossible to take the time to explain in the videotape, such as the theory and principles; these can only be explained in the book. It cannot be denied that under the tutelage of a master you can learn more quickly and perfectly than is possible using only tapes and books. What you are missing is the master's experience and feeling. However, if you ponder carefully and practice patiently and perseveringly, you will be able to make up for this lack through your own experience and practice. This book and the tape are designed for self-instruction. You will find that they will serve you as a key to enter into the field of Qigong.

References

1. "Life's Invisible Current," by Albert L. Huebner, *East West Journal,* June 1986.

2. *The Body Electric,* by Robert O. Becker, M.D. and Gary Selden, Quill, William Morrow, New York, 1985.

3. "Healing with Nature's Energy," by Richard Leviton, *East West Journal,* June 1986.

4. *A Child is Born,* by Lennart Nilsson, A DTP/Seymour Lawrence Book, 1990.

5. 解剖生理學 *(A Study of Anatomic Physiology)*，李文森編著。華杏出版股份有限公司。 Taipei, 1986.

6. *Grant's Atlas of Anatomy,* James E. Anderson, 7th Edition, Williams & Wilkins Co., 9-92, 1978.

7. "Complex and Hidden Brain in the Gut Makes Stomachaches and Butterflies," Sandra Blakeslee, *The New York Times,* January 23, 1996.

8. *Bioenergetics,* by Albert L. Lehninger, pp. 5-6, W. A, Benjamin, Inc. Menlo Park, California, 1971.

9. *Photographic Anatomy of the Human Body,* by J. W. Rohen, 邯鄲出版社，Taipei, Taiwan, 1984.

10. "Restoring Ebbing Hormones May Slow Aging," by Jane E. Brody, *The New York Times,* July 18, 1995.

11. 莊子曰：〝真人之息以踵，眾人之息以喉。〞

12. 人生七十古來稀。

13. 一百二十謂之天。

14. Before birth, you have no Qi of your own, but rather you use your mother's Qi. When you are born, you start creating Qi from the Original Essence (Yuan Jing) that you received from your parents. This Qi is called Pre-Birth Qi, as well as Original Qi. It is also called Pre-Heaven Qi (Xian Tian Qi) because it comes from the Original Jing that you received before you saw the heavens (which here means the sky), i.e., before your birth.

15. 形不正，則氣不順。氣不順，則意不寧。意不寧，則氣散亂。

16. 李清庵詩云：〝調息要調無息息。〞

17. 廣成子曰：一呼則地氣上升，一吸則天氣下降，人之反覆呼吸於蒂，則我之真氣自然相接。

18. 唱道真言曰：一呼一吸通乎氣機，一動一靜同乎造化。

19. 黃庭經曰：呼吸元氣以求仙。

20. 伍真人曰：用後天之呼吸，尋真人呼吸處。

21. 靈源大道歌曰：元和內運即成真，呼吸外求終未了。

22. 大道教人先止念，念頭不住亦徒然。

23. 意不在氣，在氣則滯。

24. 孔子曰：先靜爾后有定，定爾后能安，安爾后能慮，慮爾后能得。

CHAPTER 2

What is Arthritis?
何謂關節炎？

In this chapter, we will first describe arthritis from the point of view of both Western medicine and Chinese medicine. In the second section, we will review the structure of joints so that you will more easily understand our discussion of the different forms of arthritis in the third section. In the fourth section we will briefly consider the possible causes of arthritis. Finally, in the fifth section we will review other means of preventing or curing arthritis.

2-1. WHAT IS ARTHRITIS? 何謂關節炎？

Although both the Western and the Chinese systems of medicine describe arthritis in very similar ways, especially in regards to symptoms, there are a number of differences in how the two cultures approach the disease.

The Western Viewpoints About Arthritis 西方對關節炎之看法

Before discussing arthritis, we would first like to mention another popular, non-medical term, rheumatism, which is commonly confused with arthritis. Rheumatism has come to mean so many things to so many people that it is almost impossible to give it a clear definition. The term rheumatism commonly refers to any of several pathological conditions of the muscles, tendons, joints, bones, or nerves, characterized by discomfort and disability. This includes variable, shifting, painful inflammation and stiffness of the muscles, joints, or other structures.

The term arthritis is also commonly misused to refer to any vague pain in the area of the joints. However, joints are complicated mechanisms made up of ligaments, tendons, muscles, cartilage, and bursae, and pain in them can have many different causes. Arthritis is specifically an inflammation of the joints. The word arthritis is derived from the Greek words *arthron* (joint) and *itis* (inflammation). Therefore, if you have pain or swelling caused by injury to the ligaments or muscles, it is not necessarily classified as arthritis. You can see that while arthritis is (in a popular sense) a form of rheumatism, rheumatism is not necessarily arthritis.

The symptoms or characteristics of arthritis are pain, swelling, redness, heat, stiffness, and deformity in one or more joints. Arthritis may appear suddenly or gradually, and it may feel different to different people. Some patients feel a sharp, burning, or grinding pain, while others may feel a pain like a toothache. The same person may feel it at some times as pain, and at other times as stiffness. If we look more closely at these signs we can detect certain characteristic physiological changes. These changes include dilation of the blood vessels in the affected area and an increase of blood flow at the site of inflammation. In addition, there is increased permeability in these vessels, as white blood cells, that fight infection, infiltrate the diseased tissue. Finally, fluid from the blood can also leak into the tissue and generate edema or swelling. For these reasons, arthritis may affect not only the joints, but also other connective tissues of the body. These tissues include several supporting structures such as muscles, tendons, and ligaments, and the protective coverings of some internal organs.

Depending on where and how the problem started, and on what pathologic process is operating, arthritis can be classified into different forms such as gout, osteoarthritis, rheumatoid arthritis, and many others. We will discuss these in the third section.

The Chinese Viewpoints About Arthritis 中國對關節炎之看法

Although the symptoms of arthritis remain the same everywhere, the Chinese physicians consider them from a different point of view. Like all other cases of illness, Chinese physicians diagnose by evaluating the imbalance of Qi (which the West now calls bio-electricity) in the body, as well as by considering the actual physical symptoms.

Chinese medicine has found that, before a physical illness occurs, the Qi becomes unbalanced. If this Qi imbalance is not corrected, the physical body can be damaged and the physical symptoms of sickness will appear. The reason for this is very simple. Every cell in your body is alive, and in order to stay alive and functioning, each requires a constant supply of Qi. Whenever the supply of Qi to the cells becomes irregular (or the Qi "loses its balance"), the cells start to malfunction. Chinese physicians try to intercept the problem before there is any actual physical damage, and correct the situation with acupuncture, herbal treatments, or a number of other methods. In this way they hope to prevent physical damage, which is considered the worst stage of an illness. Once the physical body, for example an internal organ, has been damaged, it is almost impossible to make a complete recovery. This approach is the root of Chinese medicine.

Chinese physicians try to diagnose arthritis in its earliest stages, before there is any physical damage. When the Qi starts to become unbalanced, although there are no physical changes, the patient suffers from nerve pain. Because human Qi is strongly affected by the natural Qi present in clouds, moisture, and the sun (both day and night), the body's Qi is easily disturbed by changes in the weather, and arthritis patients will usually feel pain in the joints. When cloud cover is low and there is a lot of moisture in the air, the potential of the earth's electromagnetic field is also increased, and your body's Qi balance can be significantly influenced. The other obvious symptom of this influence is emotional disturbance. In the West, as long as there is no symptom of physical damage, these feelings of physical and emotional pain are usually ignored, although sometimes drugs are prescribed to stop the pain. Although Western physicians sometimes consider this an early stage of arthritis, Chinese physicians do not, and refer to it instead as "Feng Shi" (風濕), or "wind moisture." This refers to the cause of the pain that the patients feel. Eastern medical dictionaries often translate "Feng Shi" as "rheumatism."

Although countless arthritis patients regularly feel their pain worsen when the weather changes, scientists who conducted studies in an experimental climate chamber at the University of Pennsylvania concluded that there is no evidence that the weather affects arthritis.[1] I believe that this is solely because Western medicine does not take Qi/bioelectricity into account. When Western medicine starts to understand the relationship between environmental Qi and human Qi, then ample evidence of this association will emerge.

In China, when Feng Shi occurs, people will usually seek out a physician to correct the problem through acupuncture, massage, acupressure, herbal treatment, Qigong exercises, or most commonly a combination of these methods. The specific treatment would, of course, depend upon the symptoms of each individual case. For example, if the Feng Shi stems from an old joint injury, the treatment will be different than if it were caused by weak joints. The key to treatment is finding the root of the Qi imbalance and correcting it. Only when this root cause is removed will the patient recover completely.

There are many possible causes of Feng Shi. The most common cause is a joint injury that never completely healed and caused a gradually increasing disturbance of the Qi circulation. Fortunately, if the patient practices the correct Qigong exercises, the joint can be healed completely and its strength rebuilt. Exercise stimulates the Qi and increases its circulation, which removes stagnation and blockages and lets the body's natural healing mechanism operate. Smooth Qi circulation is the root of health and the foundation of healing.

Feng Shi will frequently also be found in patients who were born with weak joints or deformities, such as having one leg significantly longer than the other. Naturally, the most common and serious cases of Feng Shi are caused by aging. As we grow older, the muscles and tendons degenerate and start functioning less effectively around the joints, a process that places more pressure on the cartilage, synovium (joint surface), capsule, and the bones. This is the main cause of arthritis in older people.

If a person with Feng Shi does not seek to correct the problem, or the physician fails to correct it, the Feng Shi may develop into an infectious joint problem (Guan Jie Yan, 關節炎), which is what the Chinese call arthritis, and the joint will begin to suffer physical damage. The indications of an infectious problem are swelling, redness, pain, stiffness, sometimes fever, and deformity of the joint. This stage is already considered serious. Unlike Western medicine, traditional Chinese medicine does not differentiate among the various forms of arthritis, such as gout and osteoarthritis.

Now that you have a general idea of the different viewpoints about arthritis from both the Western medicine and Chinese medicine, we will review the structure of a joint so that you will gain a clear understanding when we discuss the different forms of arthritis.

2-2. THE STRUCTURE OF JOINTS 關節的結構

It is very important that you understand the different parts which make up a joint, so that we can pinpoint exactly where the problem is.

Generally speaking, a joint is a junction where two bones meet in a way that permits each to move in relation to the other. The human body has 68 joints. Joints are made up of bones, cartilage, capsule, synovium, and ligaments. Covering the joints are tendons, muscles, and skin. Arthritis is associated mainly with cartilage, capsule, synovium, and ligaments, so we will only discuss these parts and how they function.[1]

1. **Cartilage (Figure 2-1):** 軟骨
   Cartilage, also called "gristle," is a smooth, glistening, very tough, white fibrous connective tissue attached to the surfaces of bones at the joint. It is a major constituent of the fetal and young vertebrate skeleton; with maturation it is largely converted to bone. Between cartilages is an area called "joint space" or "synovial cavity." This space contains the synovial fluid, which lubricates the cartilage and the joint space to maintain easy movement.

2. **Capsule (Figure 2-2):** 軟骨囊
   The capsule is a bag or wrapping of soft tissue that surrounds the cartilage and the joint space. The capsule is usually quite loose, which allows the joint to move easily. Within the bag is a very critical structure called the "synovium."

3. **Synovium (Figure 2-2):** 滑膜
   The synovium or "synovial membrane" is a wet, velvety, and very delicate lining on the inner surface of the fibrous capsule. It constitutes the actual "sliding surface" of the joint. It manufactures the "synovial fluid," which lubricates the joint, and also removes bits of foreign tissue, bacteria, and other waste matter from the joint space, absorbing them into the cells of the synovial lining and digesting them.

4. **Ligaments (Figure 2-3):** 韌帶
   A ligament is a band or sheet of tough, firm, compact, fibrous tissue, that closely binds the related structures, such as bones, organs, fascia, or muscle together. The ligaments at the joints hold the bones together and keep them in the correct orientation to each other. Ligaments are firm rope-like structures on the outside of the joints. Collagen, a fibrous protein, is an important component of ligaments, and is also part of the structure of bones. Collagen fibers from the ligament extend into the collagen of the bone where the two meet. However, there is a sharp change in the nature of the tissue. Collagen in bone is calcified and still, while in the ligament the collagen is not calcified, so it is relatively flexible, though still firm. Usually, when an ankle is sprained, it is the ligament that is torn or damaged, often at the place where it joins the bones.

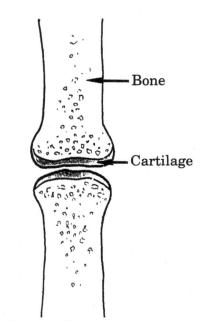

FIGURE 2-1. BONE, CARTILAGE

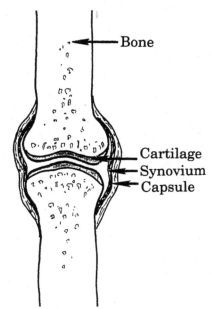

FIGURE 2-2. BONE, CARTILAGE, CAPSULE
AND SYNOVIUM

Now that you have a better understanding of the structure of a joint, let us review the different forms of arthritis and related disorders according to Western medicine.

2-3. THE DIFFERENT FORMS OF ARTHRITIS AND RELATED DISORDERS
不同形式的關節炎與有關的病症

As mentioned previously, Chinese medicine does not differentiate between the various forms of arthritis, as does Western medicine. Western medicine considers arthritis to be not a single disease, but a family of more than 100 separate diseases and disorders. Generally, they are classified according to the cause, the location of the joint where the arthritis started, and even the age of the patient. This seems

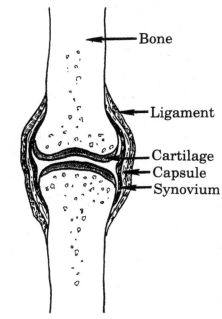

FIGURE 2-3. BONE, CARTILAGE, CAPSULE, SYNOVIUM,
AND LIGAMENT

to indicate that Western medicine has studied—or at least catalogued—the condition more deeply than have the Chinese. Let us review the most common forms of arthritis, and describe briefly how they are treated by Western medicine.

1. Infectious Arthritis: 傳染性關節炎

Infectious arthritis is generally caused by bacterial infection inside a joint (often called a "septic joint").[2] The infected joint is usually painful and may also be swollen. This form of arthritis can develop from a penetrating wound that damages the joint or from an injury in the joint area. In addition, bacteria from various infectious diseases such as tuberculosis, brucellosis, undulant fever and others may reach the joints through the blood stream and attack them. For example, arthritis can occur because of gonorrhea (a venereal disease with inflammation of the genital organs), in which the germs are carried from the infected, pus-containing genital organs through the blood to the joints.

Treatment with penicillin and other modern antibiotics is usually very successful if started promptly. Therefore, it is very important to see a physician when a joint hurts or becomes hot, swollen, or reddened; the presence of fever increases the urgency of the need for medical attention.

2. Gout: 痛風性關節炎

Gout, also called "gouty arthritis," is commonly considered to be an illness of the rich which is attributed to high living, rich food, and excessive wine (Figure 2-4). Medically, gout is considered to be an inherited ailment related to abnormal metabolism, and resulting from the retention of uric acid. Uric acid is a breakdown product of purines, which are important compounds that exist in foods such as meat and red wines; so it is a normal ingredient of the diet.

Our bodies manufacture uric acid in the liver. Whenever there is an excessive amount of uric acid, it is excreted mostly through the kidneys. If excretion is slower than production, the level of uric acid in the body can rise. This can result in gout, or in gouty lumps in bone, cartilage, or skin that are called tophi.

When excess uric acid is deposited in the joints, it may result in an inflammatory reaction from the joint tissues that causes severe pain, swelling, and stiffness (Figure 2-5). Gout attacks more men than women, commonly in the lower extremities, especially the big toes. However, any other joint in the body can also be involved (Figure 2-6). If gout is not treated promptly, it can be severe and disabling, and may lead to permanent deformity. In addition, uncontrolled gout can injure the kidneys, usually through the formation of stones.

Gout is a form of arthritis that can be effectively treated. Although certain foods may precipitate gout attacks, modern medical treatment will usually make it unnecessary to ban many "rich" foods from the diet, with the possible exception of such items as anchovies, sweetbreads, liver, and kidney. In fact, in most cases it was not the rich foods that caused the excess of uric acid in the body.

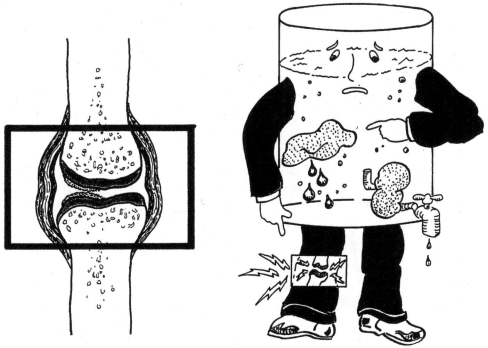

FIGURE 2-4. GOUT

FIGURE 2-5. IMBALANCED FUNCTION OF LIVER
AND KIDNEYS

Today, excellent medicines are available that can not only relieve the agony of gouty arthritis once an attack has begun, but can also prevent attacks. There are two common ways of preventing the attacks of gout through reducing the body's burden of uric acid. The first way is to block the manufacture of the enzyme that converts materials into uric acid, so that uric acid is not formed. The second way is to facilitate uric acid excretion, and thus reduce

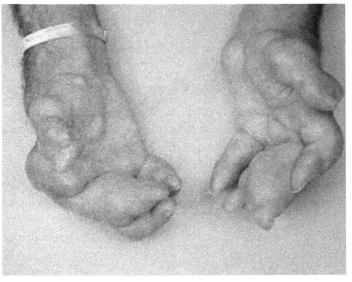

FIGURE 2-6. GOUT IN THE FINGERS

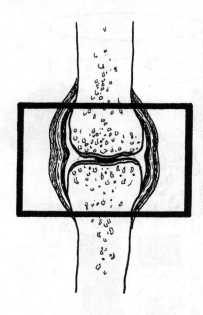

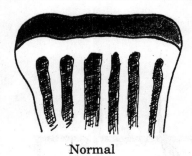

Normal

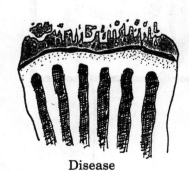

Disease

FIGURE 2-7. OSTEOARTHRITIS NORMAL DISEASE   FIGURE 2-8. NORMAL AND DISEASED CARTILAGE

the acid level. The regular use of those two methods, either together or separately, can produce gradual dissolution of the tophi and may totally prevent arthritis.

However, when an attack has already started, the drug colchicine can stop the attack, usually within twenty-four hours. Phenylbutazone and other agents may be used once an attack has started.

3. Osteoarthritis: 骨關節炎

Osteoarthritis is also called "degenerative joint disease" or "wear and tear" arthritis, and is one of the most common disorders of the human race, especially for those who are moving into old age (Figure 2-7). About 8.7% of the adult population has osteoarthritis, while only about 1% has rheumatoid arthritis. Osteoarthritis rarely develops before a person reaches forty years of age. However, X-rays show that virtually everyone over age 60 has some signs of it. X-rays taken for heart and lung conditions usually also show a touch of arthritis in the spine. However, the majority of people who show osteoarthritis in the X-rays may never experience the symptoms of aches, pain, or stiffness.

Osteoarthritis is primarily caused by repeated or prolonged microtrauma, or the repeated ignoring of minor joint injuries. When osteoarthritis attacks, it affects the cartilage of the joint, causing it to fray, wear, tear, and ulcerate. In serious cases, cartilage may split, and fragments may fall off and finally disappear entirely, leaving a bone-on-bone joint (Figure 2-8). Underneath the diseased portion of cartilage, bone may proliferate and become hard and dense. When this happens, spurs or little lumps may form on the bone at the edges of the joint (Figure 2-9). These symptoms commonly direct physicians to the diagnosis of osteoarthritis. These lumps usually do not cause discomfort to the patient.

Osteoarthritis lumps usually appear in the joints of the last section of the fingers (known as Heberden's nodes) (Figure 2-10). Pain may occur in the beginning, and then disappear after a few months. When this occurs, although the remaining lump is disfiguring, the patient can perform almost any activity without feeling discomfort.

Another common site for osteoarthritis is the neck, often due to an impact injury. Osteoarthritis also develops frequently in the lower back, the hips, and the knees. The hips and knees are especially vulnerable to osteoarthritis in overweight people, perhaps due to the extra weight bearing on the joints. X-rays show that normal knees have a wide joint space and sharp bone edges (Figure 2-11). However, in serious cases of osteoarthritis, because of the loss of cartilage, the joint space is decreased and the bone is rough and condensed (Figure 2-12).

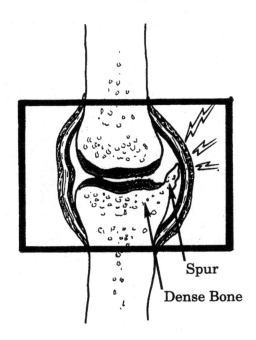

Spur

Dense Bone

FIGURE 2-9. SPURS CAN FORM ON THE BONE

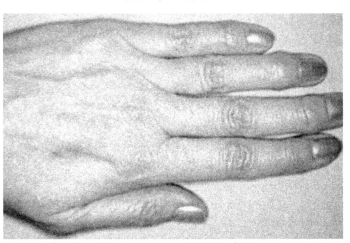

FIGURE 2-10. LUMPS OR HEBERDEN'S NODES

Although osteoarthritis usually does not result in crippling, disability may occur when severe osteoarthritis occurs in the hip. Often, the swelling and pain have a tendency to disappear after a year or so, even though X-rays may show that the arthritis becoming progressively worse.

In the last three decades, surgical techniques have been developed for hip osteoarthritis. The procedure, replacement arthroplasty, involves total hip replacement by an orthopedic surgeon. Technically, the top of the thigh bone (known as "the head of the femur") is replaced with a steel ball on a stem. The cup of the pelvis (known as the "acetabulum") is replaced with a high-density polyethylene cup. Both of the implants are secured to the living, normal bone with a fast-hardening methylmethacrylate glue-like substance (Figure 2-13). Results are very impressive. However, because the operation is relatively new, it is impossible to predict the long-term results. Similar operations have now been developed for the knees.

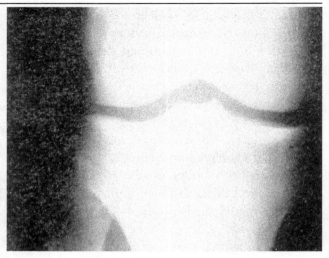

FIGURE 2-11. X-RAY OF NORMAL KNEE

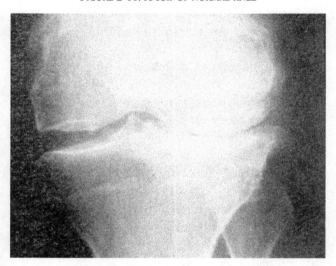

FIGURE 2-12. X-RAY OF OSTEOARTHRITIC KNEE

In Western medicine, the measures of relief from discomfort are usually provided by physicians. Treatment during the painful period may involve a variety of non-steroidal drugs or aspirin; rest and special muscle-strengthening exercises are recommended. Sometimes, an orthopedic specialist may be needed to decide if a condition of severe osteoarthritis requires special braces, exercises, or even surgical intervention.

4. Rheumatoid Arthritis: 風濕性關節炎

Rheumatoid arthritis is a chronic inflammatory disease whose cause is still not clear (Figure 2-14), but may relate to disorders of the microcirculation of blood in the joint itself. Rheumatoid arthritis affects people of all ages, and it may first appear in six-month-old babies or 60 year-old adults. The mean age of onset is around 30 to 40.

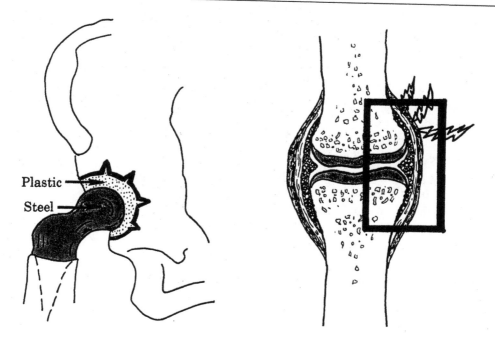

FIGURE 2-13. HIP JOINT REPLACEMENT FOR OSTEOARTHRITIS

FIGURE 2-14. RHEUMATOID ARTHRITIS

Rheumatoid arthritis usually affects up to 15 or more joints at the same time, although in one form of the disease called "monoarticular rheumatoid arthritis" only one joint is affected.

The major problems for the patient with rheumatoid arthritis are joint destruction and pain. Different from many other forms of arthritis, rheumatoid arthritis has alternating periods of remission, when the symptoms disappear, and exacerbation, marked by the return of stiffness and pain. Typically, the disease can be active for months or years, then abate, sometimes permanently. It is still not known what causes the remission, though it is not believed to result from treatment.

Many tissues may be involved in the rheumatoid process, including the lungs, spleen, skin, and occasionally the heart. However, the primary target of rheumatoid arthritis is the synovium, the joint lining. This tissue, which should be smooth and velvety, becomes inflamed, rough, granulated, and swollen. Under the microscope, cells such as lymphocytes, plasma cells, and macrophages, all elements of the body's immune or disease-fighting apparatus, are visible in samples of the tissue. It is uncertain why they are there. The unusual presence of these cells is one of a series of clues that have led to a theory that rheumatoid arthritis may be a virus-initiated disease. It has been postulated that the synovial tissue contains an antigen, a substance that is capable of stimulating an immune reaction in which body tissues attempt to reject the antigenic material by attacking the joint. In this case, scientists think that one antigen present may be a virus. Although a virus may trigger or start this immune reaction, it is the effort of the body to reject the virus or antigen that causes pain and swelling, and results in synovial destruction.

The immunological reaction that characterizes rheumatoid arthritis appears to stimulate a second reaction within connective tissue. Connective tissue forms the supporting structure of the body. It connects and surrounds the different organs and body parts and holds them in place. After a surgical incision, healing occurs by the proliferation of connective tissue. The result is a scar. Connective tissue contains the same kind of protein—collagen—which forms much of the structure of bone and cartilage. Tissue on both sides of the wound that is restructured as fresh, new collagen is deposited there.

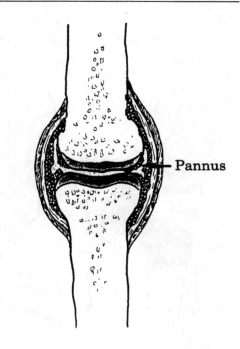

FIGURE 2-15. GROWTH OF PANNUS IN RHEUMATOID ARTHRITIS

In rheumatoid arthritis, proliferating connective or granulation tissue invades the joint cartilage. Pannus or aprons of granulation tissue grow between and across the cartilages on both bones in the joint (Figure 2-15). Pannus can also invade and destroy bone and ligaments.

The patient usually has swelling and pain in joints on both sides of the body, in a relatively symmetrical fashion. Stiffness is a major complaint, and as the disease progresses, deformities may appear. Even with very severe deformities, the joints can remain astonishingly flexible, and they are often not as painful as the deformities would suggest (Figure 2-16).

5. Juvenile Rheumatoid Arthritis: 幼年風濕性關節炎

Although rheumatoid arthritis is most common in adults, it does affect an estimated 200,000 American youngsters. Like adult arthritis, Juvenile Rheumatoid Arthritis (JRA) can sometimes begin with the swelling of many joints, although it can also begin with pain and swelling in a few joints or even a single joint. Commonly these symptoms may mistakenly be attributed to a fall or some other injury. Sometimes, before obvious signs of arthritis appear weeks or months later, JRA begins with a spiking fever, fleeting non-itching rash, and occasionally abdominal pain.

JRA is a difficult disease, but with early diagnosis and effective treatment, a relatively normal childhood can be preserved for most youngsters. Excellent functional status can eventually be regained in at least 80% of the patients, and remission (or disappearance of the disease) can occur in about two thirds of the cases. The optimal treatment for JRA, like adult rheumatoid arthritis, begins with aspirin. If aspirin is not adequate, gold salts or antimalarial drugs may be employed.

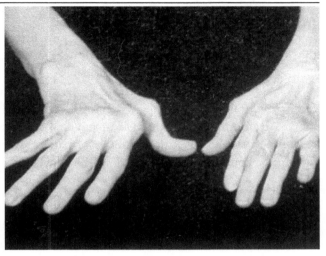

FIGURE 2-16. DEFORMITIES CAUSED BY RHEUMATOID ARTHRITIS

An exercise program tailored to the child's needs is at least as important as medication in maintaining joint function and muscle strength. For this, help from an expert physical therapist is needed. Most parents, with instruction from a therapist, become very competent cotherapists. Usually, a physician specializing in JRA is needed.

6. Ankylosing Spondylitis: 黏連性椎關節炎

Ankylosing spondylitis (AS), also referred to as "poker spine," is a special form of arthritis that affects the small joints of the spine. It affects males more often than females. Diagnosis is usually made during young adulthood. The disorder is characterized by back pain, stiffness, and loss of spinal mobility due to the involvement of spinal joints. Later these joints tend to become fused and rigid. The stiffening may sometimes extend to the ribs, limiting the flexibility of the rib cage, so that breathing is impaired. The hips and shoulders may also become inflamed and stiff.

Though AS is not fatal, it is a serious disease, and if it is not treated it can result in permanently deformed posture. In its initial stages, AS can easily be confused with many other causes of back pain. For this reason, those afflicted with the disease are frequently misdiagnosed.

The disease is usually treated with pain-relieving and anti-inflammatory drugs. The drugs may sometimes produce side effects which can be eliminated when they are withdrawn. A recent study also indicates that aspirin may be effective for some patients and should be given a trial before resorting to the other drugs. Exercise, posture training, and orthopedic correction are also important aspects of the therapy. Practice of appropriate exercises and development of constructive habits of body use in everyday activities are very helpful as AS progresses. For this reason, early recognition of the disease is important.

7. Lyme Disease: 萊姆病

This disease is caused by a tick-borne spirochete (a form of bacteria). It is now clear that Lyme disease involves many parts of the body, including the skin, the joints, the heart, and the nervous system.

The joint lesions of Lyme disease are very similar to those of rheumatoid arthritis. A recently completed study suggests that the arthritis often seen in chronic Lyme disease may have an immunogenetic basis (hereditary traits or genes that influence the immune response of the body.) Although 80% of patients may experience joint pain sometime during the course of the disease, only 10% develop chronic arthritis.

8. Lupus: 狼瘡

Systemic lupus erythematosus (SLE, or lupus) is a disorder of the body's immune system. It involves inflammation of the connective tissue, and can include arthritis when it affects the joints. The exact cause of lupus is unknown, but evidence suggests that it may result from a disorder in the body's production of antibodies (proteins that fight invading organisms).[3] In lupus, the body produces abnormal antibodies or autoantibodies that react against the patient's own tissues. Virtually every organ system can be affected, including the central nervous system. Symptoms may include psychosis, convulsions, and myelitis (inflammation of the spinal cord). A recent study has shown that normal, healthy women who have recurrent miscarriages may also have an underlying connective tissue disease such as lupus.

9. Sjogren's Syndrome: 謝格連氏病

Sjogren's syndrome and systemic lupus erythematosus are two autoimmune connective tissue diseases with distinctive, but often overlapping clinical features.[3] Sjogren's syndrome is marked by dryness of the eyes and mouth, caused by the destruction of the glands that secrete tears and saliva. It may be a primary disease, or it may be secondary to certain rheumatic diseases, such as rheumatoid arthritis, scleroderma or systemic lupus erythematosus.

10. Scleroderma: 硬皮病

Scleroderma, which literally means hard skin and is also known as progressive systemic sclerosis (PSS), is a connective tissue disorder in which excessive amounts of the protein collagen accumulate in the skin.[3] It is a disease of the vascular (blood vessel) and immune systems, as well as a connective tissue disorder. The disease can affect internal organs such as the kidneys, lungs, heart, or gastrointestinal tract and cause them to thicken and harden, which seriously affects their functioning.

11. Reiter's Syndrome: 賴透氏病

Reiter's syndrome is understood as a combination of urethritis, conjunctivitis, and arthritis.[4] This arthritis affects the spine and peripheral joints and occurs most commonly in young male adults. Usually, the first attack lasts only a few weeks or months.

Although Reiter's syndrome is not considered a venereal disease, it appears to result from infection. For example, the sexual exposure to an infectious agent can often be the cause of this disease. In addition, the disease also appears after diarrhea, sometimes during epidemics. Research has shown that most patients with the disease have a genetic predisposition to it.

12. Fibromyalgia: 纖維織炎

Fibromyalgia or fibrositis is a noninflammatory form of arthritis. It is characterized by aching and stiffness in joint and muscle areas that cannot yet be explained. Very often, the patient is tense, and usually has difficulty sleeping. Attacks may result from an injury, repeated muscular strain, prolonged mental tension, or depression. Fibromyalgia is not a destructive, progressive disease, nor is it disabling or crippling. However, it can be a debilitating problem for the patient and the misery can continue for years.

The fibromyalgia may disappear spontaneously or as a result of treatment. Although a drug known as amitriptyline (an antidepressant) has proven helpful in reducing pain, sleep difficulty, fatigue, and joint tenderness, the most effective therapy has been teaching the person to relax, to let go of neuromuscular tension, and to develop better habits of exercise and body use.

13. Polymyalgia Rheumatica: 多肌痛風濕病

Polymyalgia rheumatica usually afflicts people over the age of 50; it causes stiffness and severe aching in the shoulders and hips. Sometimes other joints ache as well, and a few may be swollen. If the disorder is not diagnosed and treated early, symptoms such as fever, fatigue, weight loss, and inflammation of the arteries may worsen. On rare occasions, the blood supply to the eye is affected, resulting in blindness.

The cause of polymyalgia is unknown. Without treatment, the disease may last for three years or more and can involve considerable pain and disability. Fortunately, the condition is dramatically relieved almost immediately with corticosteroid treatment. Prednisone is generally given; and most patients are well within days and can resume normal activities. The drug does not cure the disease, but it eliminates the symptoms. Long-term treatment is usually necessary. The disease tends to disappear after a period of months or years.

2-4. CAUSES OF ARTHRITIS 關節炎的起因

Although we understand how some forms of arthritis start, we are still in the dark about other forms. In this section we would like to summarize the known possible causes, and also contribute some ideas from Chinese medicine and Qigong.

1. Weakness of the Internal Organs: 內臟的虛弱

We already know that the condition of the internal organs is closely related to our health. According to Chinese medicine, there are five Yin organs which are considered the most important for our health and longevity. These organs are the heart, liver, lungs, kidneys, and spleen. Whenever any of these five organs is not functioning properly, sickness or even death can occur. Furthermore, all of these five organs are mutually interrelated. Whenever there is a problem with one, the others are always involved too. For example, gouty arthritis is caused by the improper functioning of the liver and kidneys.

2. Defective Genes: 人體基因的缺陷

Only recently it was reported that some forms of arthritis are caused by defective genes, that are inherited from one's parents. According to Chinese medicine, genes are considered the essence of your being. This essence is responsible for the production of hormones, from which the production of Qi can be enhanced. When this Qi is led to the brain, the spirit is raised. When all of these conversion processes are functioning normally, the immune system is strong and sickness is less likely. One of the main goals of Qigong is learning how to maintain the production of essence so the Qi can be produced efficiently. The abundant Qi can then be led to the brain for nourishment.

3. Weak Joints: 關節的虛弱

Weak joints can come from heredity or from lack of exercise. The body is a living machine, so the more you use it, the better condition it will be in. Chinese medicine believes that even if you have inherited a weak joint, it is still possible to strengthen it through Qigong. When you exercise, Qi is brought to the joint by the movement of the muscles and tendons. This will nourish the joint and rebuild it.

4. Injury: 受傷

According to modern medicine, some forms of arthritis are caused by injury to the joints. Although the injury may not be serious, it may have significant results. The injury can affect the muscles, tendons, ligaments, or even the cartilage and bone. Whenever any joint injury, even a minor one, is not treated, the normal smooth Qi circulation in the joint area will be affected. If the situation persists, the Qi imbalance can cause problems such as arthritis.

5. Aging: 老化

Aging has always been the cause of many sicknesses, including arthritis. When you are old, the Qi level in your body is low. Since your system is being deprived of the required amount of Qi, it starts to degenerate. One of the main goals of Qigong practice is learning how to slow down the aging process by building up the Qi in the body.

6. Qi Deficiency: 氣虛

Qi deficiency is responsible for many problems. It can be caused by emotional depression and sadness, which can lead the Qi inward and make the body Yin. This deprives the outer body of Qi. When this happens, you will generally feel cold. If the problem persists for a long time, the muscles and tendons will be affected by the lack of Qi, and the joints will be weakened.

Qi deficiency can have other causes, such as the weather. For example, your body's Qi is more deficient in the winter, and therefore, arthritis can be more serious then.

Qi deficiency can also be caused by working for prolonged periods in a damp area or by exposing your joints to the cold.

7. Tension: 緊張

Tension includes both mental tension and physical tension, which are related and cannot be separated. Constant mental and physical tension can increase the pressure on the joints. For example, some people are very tense and grind their teeth in their sleep, which can cause arthritis in the jaw.

Most body tension is caused by the emotional disturbance which is related to your mental reaction to stressful events. For this reason, learning how to regulate your mind is an important part of the treatment of arthritis.

2-5. OTHER POSSIBLE MEANS OF PREVENTING OR CURING ARTHRITIS
其他可能防止關節炎的方法

In addition to the ones already discussed, there are a number of other methods of preventing or curing arthritis. Although many of them are still awaiting scientific confirmation, they may be worth your consideration. However, you must understand that everybody has his or her own unique characteristics and his or her own unique inheritance. In addition to the habits and lifestyle that each person has developed, everyone's mental and physical structure is different. For example, some people are affected by allergies while others are not. What this means is that you cannot necessarily use the same method to treat different people, even when they have the same disease. Even modern Western medicine has found that the same treatment will not work equally well on all patients. Therefore, do not automatically brush off some of the treatment methods we will discuss. After all, Western medicine is only in its infancy, and it may come to understand and accept these alternative remedies.

1. Diet: 飲食控制

People who are experienced in Qigong have always understood food to be a significant influence on the condition of the Qi in the body. For this reason, diet is one of the main concerns of Chinese medicine. There is a saying: "You are what you eat." It is well known that improper diet is one of the main causes of gouty arthritis. The Chinese have found many different herbs that can ease the pain and reduce the swelling of arthritis. It has recently been discovered that protein, calories, and fats can reduce the inflammation of arthritis. Certain fish oils may interfere with the process of inflammation and therefore reduce the symptoms of rheumatoid arthritis.[5,6]

2. Change of Residence: 遷居

Since the Qi in your environment can affect the Qi in your body, arthritis sufferers should give serious consideration to this approach. If the climate where you live is too damp or too cold, it may be affecting your arthritis. It has recently been discovered that the Qi in our bodies can be significantly affected by the electromagnetic fields generated by modern technology, and therefore cause some forms of cancer. For example, people who live near high tension power lines tend to get cancer more often than those who do not. Perhaps similar environmental effects on arthritis will be found.

3. Change of Lifestyle: 改變生活態度

Your lifestyle affects how the Qi circulates in your body. If you frequently feel ill, especially mentally, you might need to change your lifestyle. How you think and how you coordinate the Qi pattern in your body with the natural Qi is very important for your health. Whenever your Qi circulation is against the "Dao" (道) (nature), you will be sick. You may find that walking for an hour or doing Qigong exercises every morning improves your Qi circulation.

4. Clothing: 衣著

What you wear also affects the Qi in your body. In the winter you must stay warm, and especially protect your joints. Joints that are left unprotected can loose Qi very quickly.

It has been discovered that many man-made fibers can adversely affect the Qi distribution and circulation in the body. For example, polyester is known to cause Qi stagnation, and to prevent the body's Qi from exchanging with the environmental Qi. You may have noticed that clothing made of polyester can accumulate a considerable charge of static electricity in the winter. This builds up an electromagnetic field and affects the Qi circulation in your body.

There are many other ways to improve the status of your arthritis. For example, it is reported that sexual activity can stimulate the adrenal glands to produce more corticosteroid, a hormone that reduces joint inflammation and pain. It is believed that sexual activity may also trigger the release of endorphins, a naturally-occurring painkilling substance.[7]

You can see from our brief discussion that, if we want to understand arthritis completely, we must remain humble and continue our study and research. Only then will we be able to reach the goal of a complete cure.

References

1. *Medicine for the Layman—Arthritis,* Clinical Center Office of Clinical Reports & Inquiries, Building 10B, Room 1C255, Bethesda, Maryland, 20892.

2. *The Complete Medical Guide,* Benjamin F. Miller, M.D., Simon and Schuster, New York, 1978.

3. *Arthritis, Rheumatic Diseases, and Related Disorders,* U.S. Department of Health and Human Services, Public Health Service, National Institutes of Health.

4. "An Overview of Arthritis and Related Disorders," *Caring,* January 1989.

5. *Arthritis and Diet,* Arthritis Foundation, 1314 Spring Street, N.W., Atlanta, GA 30309.

6. "Can Diet Relieve Arthritis," University of California, Berkeley, *Wellness Letter*, Volume 6, Issue 8.

7. "Arthritis and Your Love Life," 8, *Men's Health*, 1989.

How do the Chinese Treat
Arthritis? 中國如何治療關節炎

In the first chapter we said that the actual definition of Qigong is the study of Qi. This means that Qigong actually covers a very wide field of research, and includes the study of the three general types of Qi (Heaven Qi, Earth Qi, and Human Qi) and their interrelationships. However, because the Chinese have traditionally paid more attention to the study of Human Qi, which is concerned with health and longevity, the term "Qigong" has often been misunderstood and misused to mean only the study of Human Qi. Because so much attention has been given to Human Qi over thousands of years, the study of human Qigong has reached a very high level. Today it includes many fields such as acupuncture, herbal study, massage, cavity press, Qigong exercises, and even martial arts.

In this chapter I would like to summarize, according to my understanding, some of the methods commonly used in China to prevent arthritis, to ease its pain, and to cure it. I would then like to focus the discussion on how Qigong uses massage (including cavity press) and exercises to prevent and cure arthritis. Finally, I would like to point out the differences in how Western and Chinese medicine use massage and exercise to treat arthritis.

3-1. GENERAL CHINESE TREATMENTS FOR ARTHRITIS
中國一般治療關節炎之方法

The best way to treat arthritis is to prevent it from happening. However, if it has already occurred, then the appropriate course is to prevent it from getting any worse, and then to rebuild the strength of the joint so that it can resume functioning normally.

Generally speaking, if a case of arthritis has already reached the stage of serious physical damage, special treating is needed before any rebuilding can proceed. During the treating and rebuilding process, alleviating pain is always the first concern. In this section we will briefly discuss the theory behind several common methods for treating arthritis that have been developed in China.

1. Massage: 按摩

When done properly, massage will improve the Qi circulation in the joint area. Massage is commonly used when a patient suffers from Feng Shi (風濕) before arthritis and physical damage have occurred. At this time the Qi circulation is unbalanced, which may affect the nerves around the joints and cause pain. As mentioned earlier, Feng Shi can occur when a joint is weak or injured, or when a joint has degenerated because of aging. The pain usually increases when rain is coming on, because clouds and moisture accumulate great masses of electric charges that affect the Qi in our bodies. Pain can also occur when the joints are exposed to cold wind, which can significantly affect the Qi of the joints.

If the Feng Shi is caused by a minor injury, massage can help to heal the injury and ease the pain. The massage can usually prevent the Feng Shi from developing into arthritis, which the Chinese call "joint infection" (Guan Jie Yan, 關節炎). However, if the Feng Shi is caused by a weak joint or one degenerated because of aging, then once the pain is alleviated, Qigong exercises are necessary to rebuild the strength of the joint and prevent the Feng Shi from returning and developing into arthritis.

Massage is not used just to heal Feng Shi. It is very effective in increasing Qi circulation and easing the pain even when the joint infection (arthritis) has already become serious. However, because massage cannot reach deep enough into the body, it is not wise to rely on it for a cure.

2. Acupuncture: 針灸

Acupuncture is another method of temporarily stopping the pain and can increase the Qi circulation in the joint area to help its healing. The main difference between massage and acupuncture is that the former usually stays only on the surface, while the latter can reach to the center of the joint. One of the advantages of acupuncture is that, if the arthritis is caused by an old injury deep in the joint, it can heal the injury or at least remove some of the stagnated Qi or bruise.

In acupuncture, needles, or other newly developed means such as lasers or electricity are used to stimulate and increase the Qi circulation. Although acupuncture can stop the pain and can, to some degree, cure the arthritis, the process can be so time-consuming as to be emotionally draining. Acupuncture is an external method, and while it may remove the symptoms, it can usually heal arthritis only temporarily or only to a limited degree. Rebuilding the strength of the joint is a long-term proposition. Therefore, after arthritis patients have received some treatment, the physician will frequently encourage them to get involved in Qigong exercises to rebuild the joint.

3. Herbal Treatments: 藥療

Herbal treatments are used together with massage and acupuncture, especially when the arthritis is caused by an injury. The herbs are usually made into a paste or ground into powder, mixed with a liquid such as alcohol, and then applied to the joint. The dressing is changed every twenty-four hours.

Herbal treatments are used to alleviate pain, to increase the Qi circulation and help the healing of the injury, and to speed up the process of regrowth. Patients who work to rebuild weak joints through Qigong exercises can speed the process with herbal treatments.

4. Cavity Press: 點穴

Cavity Press (Dian Xue, 點穴) is the method of using the fingertips (especially the thumb tip) to press acupuncture cavities and certain other points (pressure points) on the body in order to manipulate the Qi circulation. Acupuncture cavities are tiny spots distributed over the entire body where the Qi of the body can be manipulated through massage or the insertion of needles. According to our new understanding of bioelectricity, these cavities are places where the electrical conductivity is higher than in neighboring areas. They are therefore more sensitive to external stimulation, and allow it to reach to the primary Qi channels.[1] Strictly speaking, cavity press (acupressure) should be discussed under massage. However, its theory is deeper and somewhat different from general massage. General massage covers a larger area of the joint, while cavity press focuses on the acupuncture cavities and certain non-acupuncture points. Normally, the power in cavity press can reach much deeper than in general massage. Furthermore, cavity press mostly uses the Qi channels to improve Qi circulation inside the joint, while general massage can enhance Qi circulation only superficially.

The theory of cavity press is very similar to that of acupuncture. There are a few differences, however: A. Acupuncture uses needles or other means of penetration such as lasers, while cavity press uses the fingertips to press the cavities; B. Acupuncture can reach much deeper than cavity press; C. Cavity press is easier and more convenient than acupuncture, which requires equipment and a higher level of training. This means that anyone can learn to use cavity press to treat arthritis after only a short period of training and some experience. However, it takes years of study to learn acupuncture; D. A patient can use cavity press on him or herself much more easily than acupuncture.

In cavity press, stagnant Qi deep in the joint is led to the surface. This improves the Qi circulation in the joint area, and reduces the pain considerably. The use of cavity press to speed up the healing of injured joints is very common in Chinese martial arts.

5. Qigong Exercises: 氣功運動

The main purpose of Qigong exercises for arthritis is to rebuild the strength of the joint by improving the Qi circulation. As mentioned earlier, traditional Chinese physicians believe that since the body's cells are alive, as long as there is a proper supply of Qi, the physical damage can be repaired or even completely rebuilt. They have proven that broken bones can be mended completely, even in the elderly. Even some Western physicians have now come to believe that damaged or degenerated joints can be returned to their original healthy state.[2]

Practicing Qigong not only can heal arthritis or joint injury and rebuild the joint; it is also known to be very effective in strengthening the internal organs. Many illnesses, including some forms of arthritis, stem from abnormally functioning internal organs. For example, gouty arthritis is caused by an improperly functioning liver and kidneys.[3]

According to Chinese medicine, almost all illnesses are caused by abnormal Qi circulation. Internal organs are the devices that produce and manage the circulation of Qi. Keeping organs healthy is the key to health and longevity, and Qigong is one of the most effective ways of doing this. Chinese physicians also believe that when the internal organs are healthy, the immune system will be healthy and the potential for resisting sickness will be high. A weak immune system is responsible for many illnesses, and is considered to be closely related to the occurrence of arthritis. For examples lupus erythematosus, rheumatoid arthritis, Lyme disease, Sjogren's syndrome, and scleroderma are all linked to a weak immune system.[3,4]

Before we discuss massage and exercise Qigong, let us first summarize the differences in how Chinese and Western medicine treat arthritis.

Summary: 總結

1. Prevention: 預防

Western medicine: 西醫 There are few documents that discuss how to prevent arthritis. It just does not seem to be considered important. Only when the symptoms of arthritis appear, treatment is started. Even if there is some joint pain and if there is no sign of arthritis in the X-rays, the physician may prescribe some medication for the pain, but other than that, he or she will all too often tend to ignore it.

Chinese medicine: 中醫 When a patient has a joint injury, Chinese physicians will first usually use acupuncture, massage, and herbal treatment to eliminate any bruises or Qi stagnation inside the joint. When the injury is almost healed, the physician will encourage the patient to do Qigong exercises to increase the Qi circulation and speed the healing. The most important effect of the Qigong, however, is to insure that all the bruises and stagnation in the joint are cleared up. This can be done only through the patient moving the joint. If this is not done, the bruises and stagnation will eventually develop into Feng Shi (風濕) and continue to interfere with smooth and balanced Qi circulation in the joint.

In China, when people start getting older and feel their bodies getting weaker, they will often start practicing some form of Qigong such as Taijiquan (太極拳) or Ba Duan Jin (八段錦) (The Eight Pieces of Brocade).[5,6] The practice helps them to keep their Qi circulating smoothly and to slow down the degeneration of their bodies. It also prevents Feng Shi and arthritis. Most people find that, in addition to strengthening their limbs, they are also able to restore their internal organs to full health, which is the key to health and longevity.

2. Stopping the Pain: 止痛

Western medicine: 西醫 Western medicine sometimes uses massage to alleviate pain, but more commonly drugs such as aspirin, prednisone, naprosyn, Motrin, colchicine, and many others are prescribed. The problem with drugs is that very often they have side effects, such as the disturbance of the gastrointestinal tract and skin rash caused by using Motrin, and the weakening or damaging of the internal organs caused by other medicines.[1] This is a very common problem in Western medicine, which will frequently cure one problem only to inflict another one on the patient.

Chinese medicine: 中醫 Acupuncture, massage, cavity press, and herbal treatments are commonly used to stop the pain. The treatments are used only to make the patient feel more comfortable, and is not considered part of the healing.

3. Healing: 治療

Western medicine: 西醫 Drugs can be effective in treating some forms of arthritis. For example, certain drugs can be used to regulate the liver and the kidneys, curing gouty arthritis. This approach can get quick results. However, the patient is then reliant on the drugs, which may eventually disturb the normal functioning of some organs.

When the arthritis has become serious, the joint can now be replaced with an artificial one. However, the long term effect of these replacement joints is still unknown.[3,4] Doctors now encourage arthritis patients to do certain exercises, often with significant results. However, documentation and more experimentation are still needed. For example, are there some forms of exercise which are harmful rather than beneficial to arthritis patients? So far, there is no established authority on this subject.

Electricity is now being used to speed up the healing of broken bones. As the West increases its understanding of bioelectricity (Qi), it is quite possible that ways will be found to use electricity to speed the healing and regrowth of arthritic joints.

Chinese medicine: 中醫 Massage, cavity press, and/or acupuncture are usually used first to increase the Qi circulation. If the arthritis is not too serious, these methods may be sufficient for a cure. However, if the arthritis has become serious, external and internal herbal treatments are also called for. The herbs taken internally help to increase the Qi circulation, remove bruises, or prevent further infection of the joint. Chinese medicine seeks to cure the cause of the arthritis. For example, if it is caused by an injury, then bruises and Qi stagnation must be cleared up. And if the arthritis is caused by degeneration due to aging, then Qigong exercises must be used to rebuild the joint and slow the degeneration.

In the next section we will discuss in more detail how massage and exercise Qigong can prevent and cure arthritis.

3-2. HOW CAN QIGONG CURE ARTHRITIS? 氣功如何治療關節炎

In Chinese medicine, the concept of Qi is used both during diagnosis and during treatment. A basic principle of Chinese medicine is that you must rebalance the Qi before you can cure the root of a disease. Only then can you also repair the physical damage and rebuild your physical strength and health. The theory is very simple. Your entire body is made up of living cells. When these cells receive the proper Qi supply, they will function normally and even repair themselves. However, if the Qi supply is abnormal, and this condition persists, then even though the cells were originally healthy, they will be damaged or changed (perhaps even becoming cancerous). In light of this basic Qi theory, let us first discuss why Qigong can be effective in curing arthritis. Then we will explain how Chinese massage and Qigong work, and finally we will point out the main differences in how Western and Chinese medicine use massage and exercise to treat arthritis.

Why Qigong is Effective for Arthritis? 為何氣功對關節炎有其療效？

1. Qigong Maintains and Increases Smooth Qi Circulation.

As mentioned earlier, the goal of Qigong healing is to reestablish a strong, smooth flow of Qi through the affected area. When this happens, the physical damage can be repaired and the strength rebuilt. Chinese physicians have always believed that as long as you are alive, physical damage to the body can be repaired through improving the Qi and blood circulation. Most Western physicians do not agree with this, and believe, for example, that the osteoarthritis caused by aging and the degeneration of the joints cannot be reversed. However, some Western physicians have changed their minds about this.[2]

2. Qigong Strengthens the Organs.

The greatest benefit of Chinese Qigong most likely lies in the training that is designed to regulate the Qi circulating in the internal organs. We know that these organs are vital, and if there is any problem with them we can become sick or even die. Regulating their Qi and keeping them healthy is a major goal of Qigong. In the more advanced Qigong practices, the training goes even deeper and is concerned with strengthening and improving the health of the organs. These practices balance the Yin and Yang Qi in the organs to slow down the aging process. Since the internal organs manage the various functions of your body, you must take care of them first if you want to slow down the aging process.

The Qi circulating in your body is the source of your life. When this circulation stops, you die. Let us look again at the source or origin of your Qi. Qi is energy, and it has to be produced from matter. As explained in the first chapter, the Chinese believe that the body contains two types of material that can be converted into Qi: one is called Pre-birth Essence, and the other Post-birth Essence. The Pre-birth Essence is inherited from your parents, while the Post-birth Essence is in the food and the air which you take in after your birth. Only in this century was it discovered that Pre-birth essence is actually the hormones produced by the endocrine glands. Since the quality and quantity of the hormones you produce depends on the inherent strength of your body, which was determined by the genes you received from your parents, Qigong practitioners used to believe that the genes were the Pre-birth Essence.

The formation of your organs is controlled by your genes. Once you are born, your organs are significantly affected by your lifestyle, which includes your thinking (emotional disturbances), food, air, and even the weather that you are exposed to. Your internal organs convert food and air into the Qi which circulates in your body. Any trouble in the internal organs will affect the production of Qi. Remember: Only when your internal organs are healthy will you have a normal supply of Qi, and only then will you be able to manage your life efficiently.

Your Qi can be affected by defects in your organs. The physical body is closely related to the Qi, and they affect each other. Whenever the Qi loses balance, its manifestation in the physical body will be abnormal. We know today that many diseases not confined to the organs are caused by the abnormal functioning of the organs. You can see that the condition of the internal organs is actually the foundation of your health and longevity.

3. Qigong Strengthens the Immune and Hormone Production Systems.

Western science knows that the body's immune system is closely related to the endocrine glands, which produce hormones. Hormones, as they are now understood, do not actually create processes. What they do, however, is cause the fundamental processes such as growth and reproduction to speed up or slow down. (The word hormone comes from the Greek word *hormikz*, which means to excite, to stimulate, or to stir up.) They also strengthen the ability of the immune system to fight diseases. For example, it is believed that the thymus gland (which is located just behind the top of the sternum) plays an important role in the body's immune system. Exactly how this happens is still not completely understood. We still do not know very much about the pineal gland in the upper back part of the brain, nor do we have a full understanding of the function of the thymus.[7] In fact, it has only recently come to be believed that hormone production is significantly related to the aging process.

Many of us know of people who were deathly sick, but who had a very high spirit and a strong desire to survive, and miraculously recovered. Both Western and Eastern religions tell of many such cases. Chinese Qigong practitioners believe that if a sick person can lead Qi to the brain through concentration or through a strong desire, he or she can evoke a powerful healing force. A possible explanation is that the stronger Qi flow activates the pineal and pituitary glands so that they generate more hormones. We now know that the most important function of the pituitary gland is to stimulate, regulate, and coordinate the functions of the other endocrine glands.[7] For this reason it is sometimes called the "master gland."

In Chinese Qigong, the Upper Dan Tian (Shang Dan Tian, 上丹田) (center of brain) is considered the center of your whole being. If you raise your spirit, which resides there, you can energize your body, generate amazing physical and mental strength, and recover more quickly from injury or sickness. Certain groups in the West have also recognized its importance as the center of the spirit—through "third eye," one is able to sense further than the physical eyes can see.

If we combine the understanding of old and new, East and West, we can conclude that what actually happens, probably because of mental concentration, is that a stronger current of bioelectricity is led to the pineal and pituitary glands to activate the production of hormones. This stimulates the entire endocrine system and causes it to function more effectively, improving healing, reproduction, and growth. If this is correct, then it is possible to begin a new era of scientific self-healing or spiritual healing. An alternative result is that we may learn how to devise electrical equipment to activate the pineal and pituitary glands to improve the effectiveness and speed of healing. Perhaps we may also be able to find the secret key to slowing down the aging process.

4. Qigong Raises the Spirit of Vitality.

The spirit is closely tied to the mind, and cannot be separated from it. In Qigong practice, the mind is considered the general in the battle against sickness. When the mind (general) has a strong will, thoroughly understands the battlefield (the body), wisely and carefully sets up the strategy (the breathing technique), and effectively and efficiently manages the soldiers (the Qi), then the morale (spirit) of the general and soldiers can be high. When this happens, sickness can be conquered and health regained.

When you use Qigong to treat your arthritis, you must first treat your mind by changing the way you look at your sickness and your life. The first thing you need to do is to stop passively accepting the negative things that have happened to you. Become more active and take charge of your life. Most basically, learn how to keep the pain of arthritis from disturbing your peace of mind. Remember, doing something is better than doing nothing.

Second, you must rebuild your confidence in your ability to treat your arthritis. Even though you may have failed before, don't let that discourage you. Learn about the causes of your problem, understand the theory of this new treatment, and try to think about how you can make the treatment more effective. Once you have done this, you will have rebuilt your confidence not only in the treatment, but also in your life.

Once you have built up your confidence, the third thing you need to do is to develop the willpower, patience, and perseverance needed to keep up the treatment. The best way to prevent the arthritis from returning once you have cured it is to make Qigong part of your life.

Fourth, after you have practiced Qigong for a while, you will understand your body better and you will know how to deal with the problems more easily. You may realize that the pain is not necessarily all bad. Pain draws your attention to your body and helps you to understand yourself better. Pain can also help you to build up willpower and perseverance. However, you must first know what pain is, only then will you know how to stop it. This is called "regulating your mind." Remember that medication is only a temporary solution.

You can see that Chinese Qigong heals by going to the root of the problem. It improves the entire body, both mentally and physically, and strengthens the immune system. Only when this is accomplished will the illness be healed completely. Now that you understand why Qigong can cure arthritis, let us discuss how Qigong reaches this goal.

How Can Qigong Exercises Cure Arthritis and How Are They Different From Western Arthritis Exercises?

氣功如何治療關節炎？氣功關節炎治療運動與西方關節炎治療運動有何不同？

You probably already know that Western physicians recommend exercise for arthritis, and that many books and reports of experiments have been published.[8-13] Regardless of whether or not you are familiar with these exercises, you should first understand the differences between the exercises used by Chinese Qigong and the exercises which are recommended by Western arthritis physicians. Then your mind will be clear, and you will be able to practice effectively.

First let us review the basic theory of the arthritis exercises used in the West that have proven effective. Naturally, there is no doubt that many of these theories, and even some of the practices are consistent with those of Chinese Qigong.

According to the Western conception, the key to healing arthritis is that the patient must learn how to balance exercise and rest. This means that without exercise there is no hope of healing, but too much exercise will worsen the arthritic condition. Therefore, since each individual has his or her own body and specific arthritic conditions, they must first understand their condition and then use common sense to regulate their lifestyle and exercise.

Western medicine believes that exercise has several benefits for the physical body: A. It increases the strength and flexibility of the muscles and ligaments surrounding the joints; B. It maintains or increases bone strength; C. Some active types of exercises such as long distance walking and swimming have important effects on the heart that can promote increased endurance and circulation and fight deterioration of the arteries. It is believed that even a small amount of exercise will help the patient overcome fatigue.

The basic Western theory of how exercise is able to heal arthritis is very simple. Every tissue in your body requires nutrition to work normally and effectively, and most tissues have arteries to carry these requirements to them. However, the situation is quite different for the joint cartilage. In the joints, movement is the only way that nourishment can be brought by the synovial fluid to the cartilage and that waste products can be removed. This means that exercise promotes good joint nutrition.

According to their different purposes, there are three general types of exercise recommended by Western physicians. The first type is stretching. Usually this type of exercise is designed to maintain and improve joint mobility, and consequently it decreases pain and improves function. In this type of exercise, the joint is moved or stretched as far as it will comfortably go and then pushed a little further to just past the point where pain or discomfort begins.

The second type of exercise is to increase muscle strength and consequently lend stability to vulnerable joints. However, the exercises designed for this purpose should minimize stress on the joints to avoid further injury. Therefore, many of these exercises are designed to extend and contract the muscles without moving the joints. An example of this is squeezing the fists tight and then relaxing them.

When the joint has partially recovered, the third step is to insure that it stays healthy. This is accomplished through endurance exercises such as walking, swimming, bicycling, jogging, or dancing to promote cardiovascular fitness. An ideal arthritis exercise program should include all three types.

You can see from this review how Western arthritis exercises are able to treat arthritis. What, then, are the differences between it and Chinese Qigong?

1. From the theoretical point of view, Qigong originates from the concept of regulating the Qi (from an imbalanced condition into a balanced one) both before and after any physical damage has occurred. Western medicine, however, does not yet fully accept the existence of Qi or bioelectricity, and is therefore not concerned with it.

2. Chinese Qigong considers the regulation of the body to be the most basic and important factor in successful practice. Regulating the body means to bring your body into a very relaxed, centered, and balanced state. Only then can your mind be calm and comfortable. When the body is relaxed, the Qi can circulate freely and be led easily anywhere you wish, such as to the skin or even deep into the bone marrow and the internal organs. To cure arthritis, you have to be so relaxed that you can lead the Qi deep into the joint where it can repair the damage. Western arthritis exercises are not usually specifically concerned with relaxation.

   The first priority in Qigong exercises for arthritis is learning how to relax and avoid muscle/tendon tension and stress in the joint area, which is especially critical in severe cases of arthritis. Chinese physicians reason that exercises that tense the muscles and tendons will inhibit the Qi circulation from going deep into the damaged joint. Furthermore, tension of the muscles and tendons increases pressure on the joint and can increase the damage. Therefore,

Chinese physicians recommend relaxed, gentle movements first to smoothly increase the Qi circulation. Only when the patient has rebuilt the strength of the joint will the muscles and tendons be exercised. After all, strong muscles and tendons are what will prevent future joint damage.

3. With Qigong, in addition to the body being relaxed, the breathing must be long, deep, and calm. According to Qigong theory, breathing is the strategic part of your practice. When you exhale, you instinctively and naturally lead Qi to the surface of your body, and when you inhale you lead it inward to the bone marrow and the internal organs. In Qigong, you have to learn to breathe deeply and calmly in coordination with your thinking. This way your mind can lead the Qi strongly into the damaged area. In Western arthritis exercises, only a few reports even mention breathing.[8]

4. In the first chapter we explained that since the mind is one of the major forces (EMF) of Qi or bioelectric circulation, it has an important role in healing. In order to make your Qigong practice really effective, and in addition to regulating your body and breathing, you must also regulate your mind. Regulating your mind means to lead it away from outside distractions and turn it toward feeling what is going on inside your body. In order to lead Qi to the damaged places in your body, your mind must be calm, relaxed, and concentrated so that you can feel or sense the Qi. The mind, therefore, plays a very important role in Qigong. Western arthritis exercises, on the other hand, are usually not concerned with the mind at all.

5. Another significant difference between Qigong and Western arthritis exercises is that Qigong emphasizes not only healing the joints, but also rebuilding the health of the internal organs. Remember, only when the internal organs are healthy can the root of the Qi imbalance be removed and, therefore, the cause of the sickness be corrected. But Qigong is not just concerned with bringing the organs back to health, it also works to strengthen them. The Western arthritis exercises, in contrast, are not at all concerned with the health of the internal organs.

6. One of the most significant results of Qigong practice is maintaining hormone production at a healthy level, which keeps the immune system functioning effectively. In Western medicine, imbalanced hormone production is adjusted with drugs.

7. The most significant difference between Qigong and Western arthritis exercise is probably that practicing Qigong draws the patient gradually into an acquaintance with the inner energy of his or her body. Once this is experienced, patients can start to feel energy imbalances when they are just beginning, and consequently are able to correct them before physical damage occurs. In fact, this is the key to preventing most illnesses.

Although many of the movements of Qigong and Western arthritis exercises are similar, the theory of Qigong is more profound and therefore the challenge is more significant. In fact, the best way to maintain your health and rebuild your Qi and body is by understanding the theory of Qigong and starting the training.

Because this book will also introduce Qigong massage for arthritis, we would like to point out some of the major differences between Qigong massage and regular Western massage.

How Chinese Qigong Massage Differs From Western Massage
中國氣功按摩與西方按摩不同的地方

1. Chinese massage pays attention to improving the circulation of both Qi and blood, while Western massage normally emphasizes only good blood circulation and a comfortable, easy feeling.

2. In Chinese massage, the massager and the patient must communicate with each other both through touch and through deeper levels of contact. This mutual cooperation enables the massager to use his or her mind to either lead Qi into the patient or to remove excess Qi from the patient's body. Therefore, Qigong massage requires a higher level of experience and training in concentration. This means that the massage is not limited to only a physical massage, it is also a Qi massage. The most important part of this cooperation is that the patient can use his or her own mind to relax the area being massaged and make the massage more effective. Furthermore, this cooperation helps the patient to calm the mind and relax deeply into the internal organs and bone marrow, which makes it possible for the massage to regulate the Qi. In Western massage, the coordination between the massager and the patient is not emphasized.

3. Cavity press or acupressure techniques are considered Qigong massage. Like Japanese Shiatsu massage, which is derived from Chinese acupressure, finger pressure on the cavities is used to regulate the Qi circulation and to remove Qi and blood stagnation in the affected areas. To do this kind of massage effectively requires not only that the massager knows the location of the cavities, but that he or she also understands the twelve Qi channels and how to use them to remove excess Qi from affected areas and bring in nourishing Qi. It is also extremely helpful if the massager is experienced in Qigong. This kind of practice is almost completely ignored in Western massage.

After reading this you may be discouraged about the possibility of your ever using Qigong massage techniques. As a matter of fact, you do not need such a high level of knowledge to deal with arthritis. All you really need to know is the location of the cavities or pressure points around the afflicted joint and how to apply pressure with your finger. With a bit of practice you will soon learn how to regulate the Qi there. After you have gained some experience you may even wish to study Qigong massage and learn more about using it for healing. In this book we will focus only on the massage and cavity press techniques that are related to arthritis. If you are interested in pursuing the subject in more depth, read my book *Chinese Qigong Massage—General Massage.*

References

1. *The Body Electric,* by Dr. Robert 0. Becker, MD., and Gary Selden, 1985. William Marrow and Company, Inc., 105 Madison Ave., New York, 10016.

2. "Keeping the Human Body Active Reduces Risk of Osteoarthritis," by Dr. Gifford-Jones, *Globe and Mail,* Toronto, Ont., January 31, 1989.

3. *Medicine for the Layman—Arthritis,* Clinical Center Office of Clinical Reports & Inquiries, Building l0B, Room 1C255, Bethesda, Maryland, 20892.

4. "An Overview of Arthritis and Related Disorders," *Caring,* January 1989.

5. *The Essence of Taiji Qigong,* Dr. Yang, Jwing-Ming, YMAA, 1990.

6. *Eight Simple Qigong Exercises for Health,* Dr. Yang, Jwing-Ming, YMAA, 1988.

7. *The Complete Medical Guide,* Benjamin F. Miller, M.D., Simon and Schuster, New York, 1978.

8. "Use It or Lose It," Kate Lorig, R. N., Dr. P. H., and James F. Fries, M.D., *Aim Plus,* January/February, 1989.

9. "The Good News About Exercises," Peggy Person, *Arthritis Today,* May/June, 1989.

10. "How to Choose the Right Exercise," *Arthritis Today,* January/February, 1987.

11. *Understanding Arthritis,* Irving Kushner, M.D., Charles Scribbler's Sons, New York, 1984.

12. "Exercise and Arthritis," Richard S. Panush and David G. Brown, *Sports Medicine* 4: 54-64, 1987.

13. *Osteo-Arthritis,* Fred L. Savage, Station Hill Press, Barrytown, New York, 1988.

CHAPTER 4

Qigong for Arthritis
氣功治療關節炎

4-1. INTRODUCTION 介紹

Before proceeding any further, we would like first to discuss the attitude which you need to adopt in your practice. Quite frequently, people who are ill are reluctant to become involved in the healing process. This is especially true for arthritis patients. Both Western and Chinese physicians have had difficulty persuading them to become involved in regular exercise or Qigong. The main reason for this reluctance is that the patients are afraid of pain, and therefore believe that these kinds of exercise are harmful. In order to conquer this obstacle to your healing, you must understand the theory of healing and the reason for practicing. Only then will you have the confidence necessary for continued practice. Remember, a physician may have an excellent prescription for your illness, but if you don't take the medicine, it won't do you any good.

Another factor that has caused the failure of many a potential cure is lack of persistence. Because the healing process is very slow, it is very easy to become impatient and lazy. Very often in life we will know exactly what it is that we need to do, but because we are controlled by the emotional parts of our minds, we end up either not doing what we need to, or not doing it right. Either way, our efforts will have all been in vain.

It seems that most of the time our "emotional mind" and "wisdom mind" are in opposition. In China there is a proverb which says: "You are your own biggest enemy." This means that your emotional mind often wants to go in the opposite direction from what your wisdom mind knows is best. If your wisdom mind is able to overcome your emotional mind, then there is nothing that can stop you from doing anything you want. Usually, however, your emotional mind causes you to lose your willpower and perseverance. We always know that our clear-headed wisdom mind understands what needs to be done, but too often we surrender to our emotional mind and become slaves of our emotions.

The first step when you decide to practice Qigong is to strengthen your wisdom mind and use it to govern your emotional mind. Only then will you have enough patience and perseverance to keep practicing. You can see that the first key to successful training is not the techniques themselves, but rather your self-control. I sincerely believe that as long as you have a strong will, patience, and perseverance, there is nothing that you can't accomplish.

Forming the habit of practicing regularly actually represents changing your lifestyle. Once you have started regulating your life through Qigong, not only can it cure your arthritis and restrengthen your joints, but it can also keep you healthy and make both your mental and physical lives much happier.

This chapter will focus on discussing the Qigong practices I am familiar with, leaving other methods, such as acupuncture and herbs to other references. Before we discuss the actual practices, we would first like to remind you of the keys to successful practice. Only if you follow these keys in your practice will you be able to see and feel how Chinese Qigong is different from similar Western arthritis exercises.

Important Training Keys: 練習重點

1. Regulating the Body: 調身

Before you start your Qigong exercises, you should first calm down your mind and use this mind to bring your body into a calm and relaxed state. Naturally, you should always be concerned with your mental and physical centers. Only then will you be able to find your balance. When you have achieved both mental and physical relaxation, centering, and balance, you will be both natural and comfortable. This is the key to regulating your body.

When you relax, you should learn to relax deeply into your internal organs, and especially the muscles that enclose the organs. In addition, you must also place your mind on the joints that are giving you trouble. The more you can bring your mind deep into the joint and relax it, the more Qi will circulate smoothly and freely to repair the damage.

2. Regulating the Breathing: 調息

As mentioned before, breathing is the central strategy in Qigong practice. According to Qigong theory, when you inhale you lead Qi inward and when you exhale you lead Qi outward. This is our natural instinct. For example, when you feel cold in the wintertime, in order to keep from letting the Qi out of your body, you naturally inhale more than you exhale to lead the Qi inward, which also closes the pores in the skin. However, in the summertime when you are too hot you naturally exhale more than inhale in order to lead Qi out of your body. When you do this you start to sweat and the pores open.

In Qigong, you want to lead the Qi to the internal organs and bone marrow, so you must learn how to use inhalation to lead the Qi inward. When you use Qigong to cure your arthritis, you must inhale and exhale deeply and calmly so that you can lead the Qi deep into the joint and also outward to dissipate the excess or stagnant Qi that has accumulated in the joints. Therefore, in addition to relaxing when you practice, you should always remember to inhale and exhale deeply. When you inhale, place your mind deep in the joint, and when you exhale, lead the Qi to the surface of the skin.

3. Regulating the Mind: 調心

In Qigong, the mind is considered the general who directs the battle against sickness. After all, it is your mind that manages all of your thinking and activity. Therefore, a clear, calm mind is very important so that you can judge clearly and accurately. In addition, your attention must also be concentrated. Your mind can generate an EMF (an electromotive force or "voltage") that causes your Qi to circulate. The more you concentrate, the more strongly you can lead the Qi.

When you have a calm and concentrated mind, you will be able to feel and sense the problem correctly. Therefore, when you practice Qigong for your arthritis, you must learn how to bring your mind inward so that you can understand the situation, and you must know how to use your concentrated attention to lead the Qi.

4. Regulating the Qi: 調氣

Once you have regulated your body, breathing, and mind, you will be in a good position to start regulating your Qi, and will be able to lead your Qi anywhere in your body in order to make repairs.

5. Regulating the Spirit: 調神

The final key to Qigong is raising your spirit of vitality. Good morale or fighting spirit is necessary to win the struggle against illness. When your spirit is high, your willpower is strong, your mind is firm, and your patience can last a long time. In addition, when your spirit is high your emotions are under control and your wisdom mind can stimulate the Qi to circulate in the body more efficiently. This will significantly reduce the time of healing.

You should now have a clear idea of how to practice most efficiently. During the course of your practice, you should frequently remind yourself of these key requirements. If you would like to learn more about the keys to Qigong practice, you may refer to the YMAA book: *The Root of Chinese Qigong*. In the next section we will introduce several Qigong exercises that can be used to strengthen and maintain the health of the internal organs. The third section will discuss Qigong massage and cavity press for arthritis. Finally, the fourth section will introduce many Qigong exercises that can rebuild the strength of the joints.

4-2. Qigong for Strengthening the Internal Organs 氣功強健內臟

Your internal organs are the foundation of your health. Most deaths are due to the malfunction or failure of the internal organs. In order to be healthy and avoid degeneration, your organs need to have the correct amount of Qi circulating smoothly through them.

The internal organs manage the energy in our bodies, and carry out a variety of physical processes. When any organ starts to malfunction, the Qi circulation in the body will be disrupted, and the production of hormones will be affected. This state can result in a variety of disorders, including gouty arthritis.

In this section, we would like to introduce two types of Qigong practices that are commonly used to improve Qi circulation, especially around the internal organs. The first exercise is massaging the internal organs by moving the muscles inside the torso. If you would like to have more information on the theory behind this subject, please refer to my book *The Eight Simple Qigong Exercises*.

The second type of Qigong practice is improving the Qi circulation around the internal organs by massaging either directly over the organs or on acupuncture cavities that are connected to the organs. If you are interested to know about massage, please refer to my book: *Chinese Qigong Massage*.

Massaging the Internal Organs with Movement 內臟按摩運動

All of the internal organs are surrounded by muscles. Except for some of the trunk muscles that we use constantly throughout the day, most of these muscles are ignored. According to Qigong theory, if you can bring your Yi (意) (wisdom mind) to a muscle, you can lead Qi to energize it and move it. For example, if you decide you want to be able to wiggle your ears and keep trying, you will eventually be able to. It's the same with the internal muscles. This means that, if you practice becoming very calm and bringing your attention deeper and deeper into the center of your body, you will soon be able to feel and sense the structure and condition of the insides of your body. Once this happens you can use your mind to move the internal muscles and massage the internal organs.

The way to reach this goal is to start by using your trunk muscles to make the muscles deeper inside your body move. After you have practiced for a while, your mind will be able to reach deeper and feel other muscles as well. Once you are able to feel these muscles, you will be able to move them. With a bit more practice you will be able to control them while keeping them relaxed, and the movements will become natural, easy, and comfortable. Remember that the muscles have to be relaxed before the organs can be relaxed and before the Qi can circulate smoothly.

In this sub-section, we will introduce the beginning steps of internal organ massage through trunk movement. After you are able to do these exercises easily and smoothly, you should continue to lead your mind deeper and deeper into your body and sense your organs.

It is a good idea to loosen up your trunk before starting these massaging movements. This will let you move more naturally and comfortably.

Loosening the Torso Muscles 人體軀幹的放鬆

The torso is the center of the whole body, and it contains the muscles that control the torso and also surround the internal organs. When the torso muscles are tense, the whole body will be tense and the internal organs will be compressed. This causes stag-

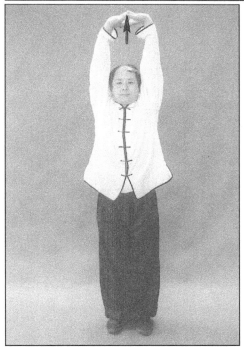

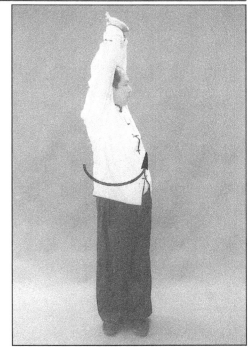

FIGURE 4-1   FIGURE 4-2

nation of the Qi circulation in the body and especially in the organs. For this reason, the torso muscles should be stretched and loosened up before any moving Qigong practice.

First, interlock your fingers and lift your hands up over your head while imagining that you are pushing upward with your hands and pushing downward with your feet (Figure 4-1). Do not tense your muscles, because this will constrict your body and prevent you from stretching. If you do this stretch correctly, you will feel the muscles in your waist area tensing slightly because they are being pulled simultaneously from the top and the bottom. Next, use your mind to relax even more, and stretch out a little bit more. After you have stretched for about ten seconds, turn your upper body to one side to twist the trunk muscles (Figure 4-2). Stay to the side for three to five seconds, turn your body to face forward and then turn to the other side. Stay there for three to five seconds. Repeat the upper body twisting three times, then tilt your upper body to the side and stay there for about three seconds (Figure 4-3), then tilt to the other side. Next, bend forward and touch your hands to the floor (Figure 4-4) and stay there for three to five seconds. Finally, squat down with your feet flat on the floor to stretch your ankles (Figure 4-5), and then lift your heels up to stretch the toes (Figure 4-6). Repeat the entire process ten times. After you finish, the inside of your body should feel very comfortable and warm.

The torso is supported by the spine and the trunk muscles. Once you have stretched your trunk muscles, you can loosen up the torso. This also moves the muscles inside your

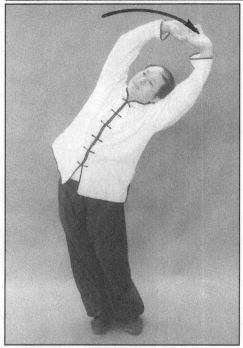

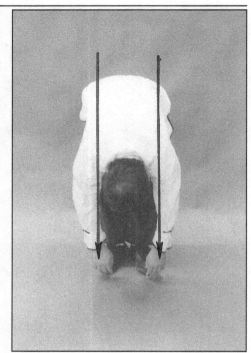

FIGURE 4-3   FIGURE 4-4

body around, which moves and relaxes your internal organs. This, in turn, makes it possible for the Qi to circulate smoothly inside your body.

a. Massaging the Large Intestine, Small Intestine, Urinary Bladder, and Kidneys
按摩大腸、小腸、膀胱、與腎臟

This exercise helps you to regain conscious control of the muscles in your abdomen. There are four major benefits to this abdominal exercise. First, when your Lower Dan Tian (Xia Dan Tian, 下丹田) area is loose, the Qi can flow in and out easily. The Lower Dan Tian is the main residence of your Original Qi (Yuan Qi, 元氣). The Qi in your Dan Tian can be led easily only when your abdomen is loose and relaxed. Second, when the abdominal area is loose, the Qi circulation in the large and small intestines will be smooth, and they will be able to absorb nutrients and eliminate waste more efficiently. If your body does not eliminate effectively, the absorption of nutrients will be hindered, and you may become sick. Third, when the abdominal area is loose, the Qi in the kidneys will circulate smoothly and the Original Essence stored there can be converted more efficiently into Qi. In addition, when the kidney area is loose, the kidney Qi can be led downward and upward to nourish the entire body. Fourth, these exercises eliminate Qi stagnation in the lower back, healing and preventing lower back pain.

To practice this exercise, stand with your feet a comfortable distance apart and your knees slightly bent. As you get more used to this exercise and your legs become stronger,

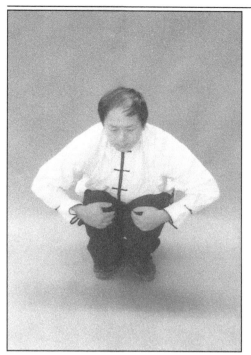

FIGURE 4-5

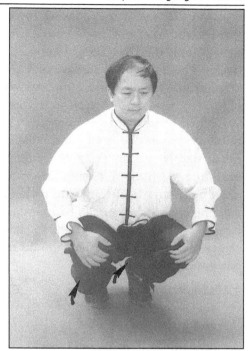

FIGURE 4-6

bend your knees a little bit more. Without moving your thighs or upper body, use the waist muscles to move the abdomen around in a horizontal circle (Figure 4-7). Circle in one direction about ten times, and then in the other direction about ten times. If you hold one hand over your Lower Dan Tian and the other on your sacrum, you may be able to focus your attention better on the area you want to control.

In the beginning you may have difficulty making your body move the way you want it to, but if you keep practicing you will quickly learn how to do it. Once you can do the movement comfortably, make the circles larger and larger. Naturally, this will cause the muscles to tense somewhat and inhibit the Qi flow, but the more you practice the sooner you will be able to relax again. After you have practiced for a while and can control your

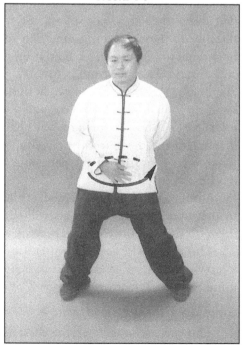

FIGURE 4-7

waist muscles easily, start making the circles smaller, and also start using your Yi to lead the Qi from the Dan Tian to move in these circles. The final goal is to have only a slight physical movement, but a strong movement of Qi.

When you practice, concentrate your mind on your abdomen, and inhale and exhale deeply and smoothly. Remember that breathing deep does not mean breathing heavily. When you breathe deep, keep the diaphragm and the muscles surrounding the lungs relaxed. Inhale to lead the Qi into the center of the body and exhale to lead the Qi out through the skin.

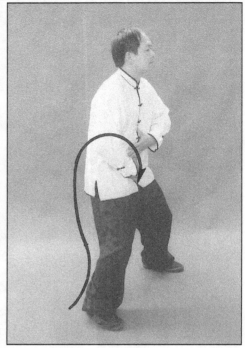

FIGURE 4-8

b. Massaging the Stomach, Liver, Spleen, Gall Bladder, and Kidneys
按摩胃、肝、脾、膽、與腎臟

Beneath your diaphragm is your stomach, to the right are your liver and gall bladder, and to the left is your spleen, and in the back are your kidneys. Once you can comfortably do the circular movement in your lower abdomen, change the movement from horizontal to vertical, and extend it up to your diaphragm. The easiest way to loosen the area around the diaphragm is to use a wave-like motion between the perineum and the diaphragm (Figure 4-8). You may find it helpful when you practice this to place one hand on your Lower Dan Tian and your other hand above it with the thumb on the solar plexus. Use a forward and backward wave-like motion, flowing up to the diaphragm and down to the perineum and back. While you do this, inhale deeply when the motion is starting at the perineum and exhale as it reaches the diaphragm. Practice ten times.

Next, continue the movement while turning your body slowly to one side and then to the other (Figure 4-9). This will slightly tense the muscles on one side and loosen them on the other, which will massage the internal organs. Repeat ten times.

This exercise loosens the muscles around the stomach, liver, gall bladder, spleen, and kidneys, and therefore improves the Qi circulation there. It also trains you in using your mind to lead Qi from your Lower Dan Tian upward to the solar plexus area.

c. Massaging the Lungs and Heart 按摩肺與心

This exercise loosens up the chest and helps to regulate and improve the Qi circulation in the lungs. According to the theory of the five phases in Chinese medicine, the

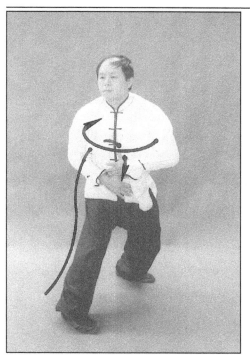

FIGURE 4-9

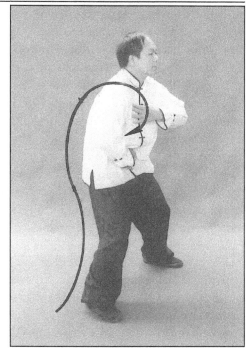

FIGURE 4-10

lungs belong to the element Metal (Jin, 金) while the heart belongs to the element Fire (Huo, 火). Metal is able to cool down Fire, and the lungs are able to regulate the Qi of the heart. The heart is the most vital organ, and its condition is closely related to our life and death. If there is too much Qi in the heart (when it is too Yang), you speed up its degeneration and become prone to heart attacks. For this reason, Qigong places great emphasis on using the lungs to regulate the Qi in the heart. If we know how to relax the lungs and keep the Qi circulating in them smoothly, they will be able to regulate the heart more efficiently.

After loosening up the center portion of your body, extend the movement up to your chest. The wave-like movement starts in the abdomen, moves through the stomach, and up to the chest. You may find it easier to feel the movement if you hold one hand on your abdomen and the other lightly touching your chest (Figure 4-10). After you have done the movement ten times, extend the movement to your shoulders (Figure 4-11). Inhale when you move your shoulders backward and exhale when you move them forward. The inhalation and exhalation should be as deep as comfortably possible, and the entire chest should be very loose. Repeat the motion ten times.

Massaging the Internal Organs with your Hands 用手按摩內臟

Using the hands to massage the internal organs is a natural human instinct, and we do it whenever we feel pain or Qi stagnation in or near an organ. For example, if you have a diarrhea and feel pain in your abdomen, you naturally massage yourself with your hand. Or if you overeat you automatically stroke or rub your stomach with your palms to ease the pain.

According to Chinese medicine, in the center of each palm is a cavity or gate called the "Laogong (P-8)" (勞宮) which is used to regulate the Qi of the heart whenever the Qi flow is too strong (Figure 4-12). Unless you are sick, the Qi in the heart is normally more positive than is necessary, especially in the summertime. When you are excited or nervous, even more Qi accumulates around the heart. When this happens, the centers of your palms will feel warm and will often sweat.

Since the Qi in the center of the palm is always strong, you can use this Qi to help the stagnant organ Qi to flow smoothly. Chinese physicians and Qigong practitioners have developed a number of ways of using the

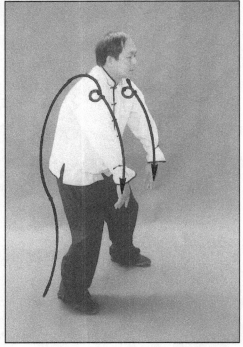

FIGURE 4-11

hands to improve the Qi circulation in the internal organs. In this section we will introduce a few common ones that can be practiced easily by anyone. It is not true that only an expert can heal people with his hands. Anyone can do it if they know how.

a. Abdomen 小腹

To massage your abdomen and regulate the Qi circulation in your large and small intestines, place one hand on top of the other on your lower abdomen (Figure 4-13). If you are right-handed, it is better if you place your right hand on the bottom and the left hand on the top. Naturally, if you are left-handed, place the left hand on the bottom. The reason for this is quite simple: the Qi is strongest in the hand you use most often, and it is easier for you to lead the Qi from it.

When you massage your abdomen, it is best if you lie down so that your lower body is relaxed and the Qi can circulate more easily and smoothly. Hold you hand lightly against the skin and gently circle your hands clockwise, which is the direction of movement within the large intestine (Figure 4-13). Circling in the other direction would hinder the natural movements of peristalsis. Massage until you feel warm and comfortable deep inside your body.

As you massage, your breathing should be relaxed, deep, and comfortable. Place your mind a few inches under your palms. The mind will then be able to lead the Qi inward to smooth out Qi and blood stagnation.

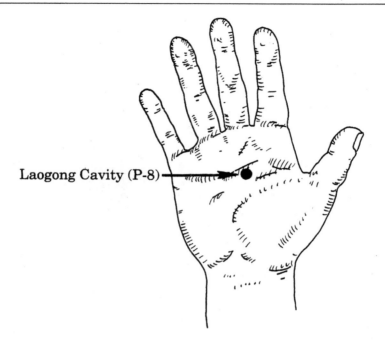

Laogong Cavity (P-8) —→

FIGURE 4-12. LAOGONG CAVITY

b. Liver, Stomach, Spleen, and Gall Bladder
肝、胃、脾、與膽

In Qigong massage for the internal organs, the liver, stomach, spleen, and the gall bladder are usually included in the same techniques because they are all located in the middle of the front of the body. Maintaining healthy Qi circulation in an organ requires not only that the circulation in the organ

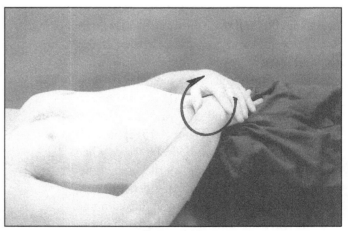

FIGURE 4-13

itself be smooth, but also that the circulation between the organs be smooth. Therefore, when you massage these four internal organs, you should treat them as one instead of four.

Hold your hands as you did when massaging the lower abdomen, only now place them above the navel. Experience has shown that clockwise is again more effective than counterclockwise (Figure 4-14). It is easiest to do this massage when you are lying down.

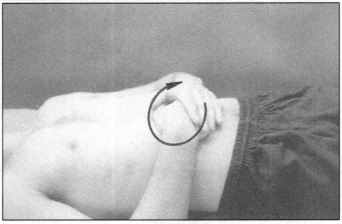

FIGURE 4-14

It is also best if you have someone else to massage you, because it is then easiest for you to relax. Massage until you feel warm inside.

c. Kidneys 腎

Chinese medicine considers the kidneys to be perhaps the most important internal organs. The kidneys affect how the other organs function, so almost all forms of Qigong place heavy emphasis on keeping them healthy.

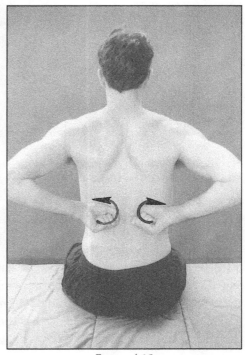

FIGURE 4-15

To massage your own kidneys, close your hands into fists and place the thumb/index finger sides on your kidneys. Gently circle both fists until the kidneys are warm. In the summer, when your kidneys are normally too Yang, it is desirable to dissipate some of the Qi. This can be done by circling your right hand clockwise and your left hand counterclockwise (Figure 4-15). This leads the Qi to the sides of your body. However, when you massage your kidneys in the wintertime, when the kidney Qi is normally deficient (too Yin), then you should reverse the direction and lead the Qi to the center of your back to nourish the kidneys. As usual, the breathing and the mind are important keys to successful practice.

There are other methods of improving the Qi circulation in the kidneys. One of the most common ones is to massage the bottoms of your feet. There is a Qi gate in the front center of each sole that is called "Yongquan

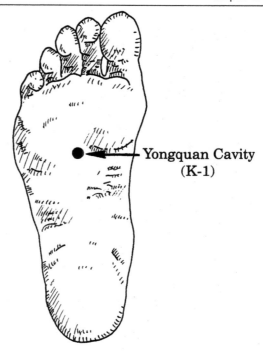

FIGURE 4-16 YONGQUAN CAVITY

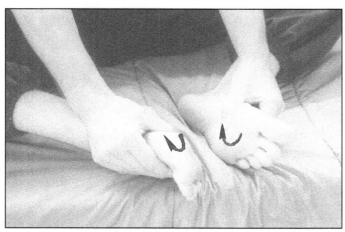

FIGURE 4-17

(K-1)" (湧泉) (Bubbling Well) (Figure 4-16). Massaging these two cavities will stimulate the Qi circulation in the kidneys and help to regulate them (Figure 4-17).

d. Lungs 肺

As mentioned earlier, in the theory of the Five Elements the lungs belong to Metal (Jin, 金) while the heart belongs to Fire (Huo, 火). According to this theory, the Metal lungs can

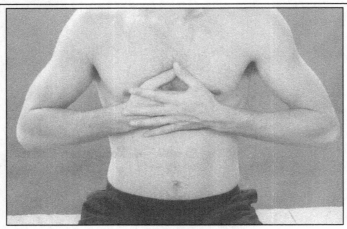

FIGURE 4-18

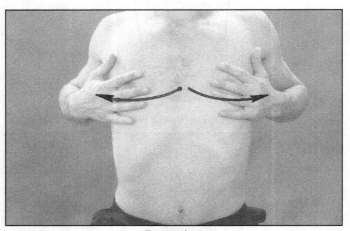

FIGURE 4-19

be used to regulate the heart Fire just as metal can absorb heat. If you pay attention careful-ly, you will notice that when you feel heat around your heart due to excitement or even depression, you will normally thrust out your chest and greatly expand your lungs while inhaling. Doing this a few times reduces the pressure and the feeling of heat in the heart.

To do Qigong massage for your lungs, place both hands on the center of your chest just above the solar plexus (Figure 4-18). Inhale deeply, and then exhale while lightly pushing both hands to the sides (Figure 4-19). Do this until your lungs feel relaxed and comfortable. This massage is also good for the heart.

e. Heart 心

Qigong teachers do not normally encourage students to massage their own hearts unless they are fairly advanced in skill. The heart is the most vital organ, and if you mis-treat it you are in big trouble.

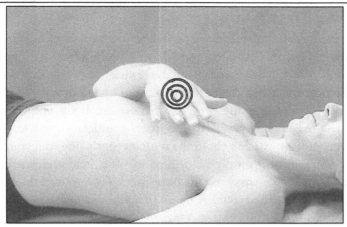

FIGURE 4-20

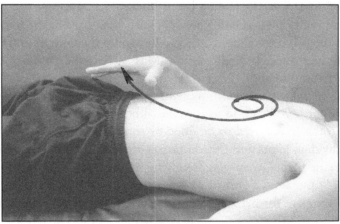

FIGURE 4-21

When you massage your heart, unlike all the other internal organs, you cannot place your mind on it. If you do place your mind on your heart, you will lead more Qi to it and make it even more positive. You may have noticed that when your heart is beating fast after exercising, if you pay attention to your heartbeat it will start beating even faster. A person who is prone to heart attacks can possibly bring one on by paying too much attention to his heart. If your heart is beating too hard, the best thing is to pay attention to your lungs and breathe deeply and gently. After only a few breaths your heart will slow down and regain its regular pace.

Therefore, when you massage your heart, your mind should not be on your heart. Instead, keep your mind on the movement of your hands. To massage your heart, place your right hand over your heart at least three inches away from your chest (Figure 4-20). Move your hand in a small clockwise circle, and gradually increase the size of the circle. This takes the Qi in the heart and spreads it out around the chest. Finally, lead the Qi by the liver and down the right leg (Figure 4-21).

f. Testicles or Ovaries 睪丸或卵巢

Massaging the testicles or ovaries increases the production of hormones. According to Chinese Muscle/Tendon Changing and Marrow/Brain Washing Qigong (Yi Jin Jing and Xi Sui Jing) (易筋經、洗髓經), massaging the testicles or ovaries correctly will increase hormone production and also increase the amount of Qi led upward to the brain. Other effects are increasing the amount of Qi stored in the body and strengthening the immune system. There are many ways to massage the testicles or ovaries. For example, if you massage your testicles, you may hold the testicles gently between your palms and circle your hands. You may also simply hold them in your hand and gently press and rub them. To massage ovaries, you may use the base knuckles of your pinkies to circle ovaries gently. This subject is discussed in more detail in my books *Qigong—The Secret of Youth* and *Chinese Qigong Massage.*

4-3. MASSAGE AND CAVITY PRESS (ACUPRESSURE) 點穴按摩

Massage and cavity press (Dian Xue, 點穴) are often used at the same time in treating arthritis. Massage is generally used first to loosen up the muscles and tendons around the joint and to increase the Qi circulation. Massage lets the power of the cavity press penetrate deeper into the joint.

In this section, we will introduce some of the more common and easy-to-learn techniques. Many of them you can do to yourself, although the majority, such as those done on the neck and the spine, need to be done by someone else. Before we discuss how to massage the individual joints and the location of the cavities, we would first like to mention one important point: when you are giving massage or cavity press treatments, you should not over-stimulate the area or cavity (pressure point). Over-stimulation can only cause pain and generate further stagnation of the Qi and blood. In addition, too much pressure can further injure a joint that may be starting to heal. The purpose of massage and cavity press is to increase the Qi and blood circulation, and anything that causes pain is incorrect. Next, we will introduce some of the basic massage and cavity press techniques.

Basic Massage and Cavity Press Techniques 基本按摩與點穴技巧

The first basic technique for massaging joints is to place a hand on the joint and rub gently back and forth or in circles until the area is warm (Figure 4-22). As the joint gets looser, you may increase the pressure as you rub so that the power penetrates deeper into the joint.

The second technique uses the middle joints of the fingers to massage. Hold the area you are massaging with the middle knuckles of your fingers, and be sure not to press the thumbs in and cause bruises (Figure 4-23). You want to feel the muscles and tendons, so apply gentle pressure and penetrate inward with your mind. Do not rub the skin. Instead, move your fingers back and forth and in circles to massage the muscles and tendons beneath the skin.

The third technique uses the thumb to rub or press and circle along the muscles and tendons of the joints (Figure 4-24). The other four fingers are usually used to stabilize

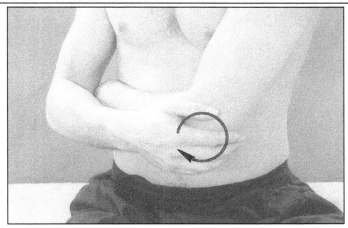

FIGURE 4-22

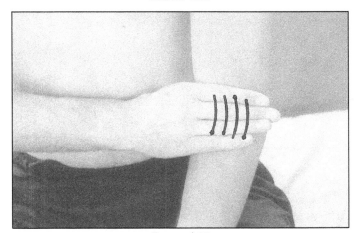

FIGURE 4-23

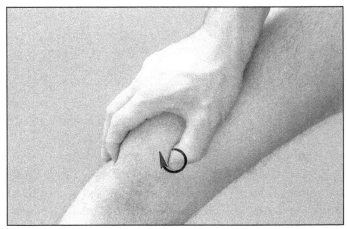

FIGURE 4-24

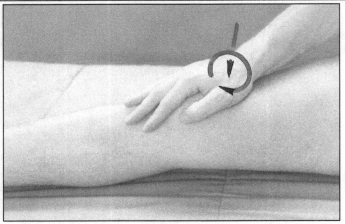

FIGURE 4-25

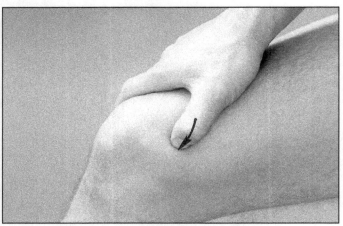

FIGURE 4-26

the thumb. This technique is used to increase the Qi circulation and to lead the Qi away from the joints.

The last basic technique uses the base of the palm (Figure 4-25). Press your palm lightly inward to touch the muscles and tendons that you want to massage, and then move your palm in circles. Do not rub the skin. After you have loosened one area, follow the muscle and tendon away from the joint and repeat the procedure. Adjust the pressure to control the depth of the massage and stimulate the various levels of muscle and tendon.

In cavity press you use a fingertip to press directly on the cavity while concentrating deeply. The thumb press (Figure 4-26) is usually used most often, and the index finger (Figure 4-27) and middle finger (Figure 4-28) are also used. Occasionally, when greater pressure is desired, the index and middle fingers are used together (Figure 4- 29). Frequently, pressure is applied with a circular motion. If you are using your right hand, a

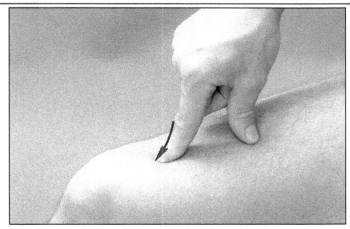

FIGURE 4-27

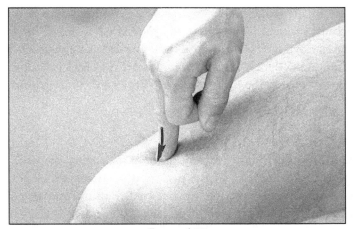

FIGURE 4-28

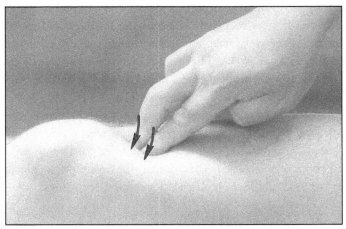

FIGURE 4-29

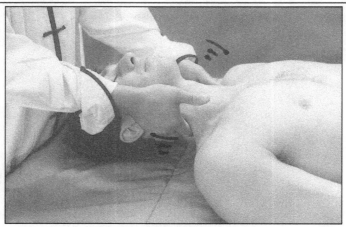

FIGURE 4-30

clockwise motion usually nourishes the cavity while a counterclockwise one lowers the Qi level. This is because a clockwise motion leads your Yi (意) (mind) forward and a counterclockwise one leads your Yi back. Naturally, if you are using your left hand, you circle counterclockwise to lead the Qi forward and clockwise to lead it backward. Remember, your Yi is the key to leading the Qi forward and backward through your fingers.

A. The Neck and Spine 頸與脊椎

a. Neck 頸部

Massage (An Mo, 按摩). The main purpose of massaging the neck is to loosen up the two main muscles in the back of the neck and to increase the Qi circulation. The best posture for a neck massage is lying on your back with the massager above your head (Figure 4-30). An alternate way is sitting with the head pushed slightly back to relax the muscles. Starting at the top of the neck, rub downward with your thumbs. You may do this yourself (Figure 4-31) or have a partner do it for you (Figure 4-32). Next, use the middle joints of your fingers to gently squeeze the muscles and move them around. Again, it is easier and more comfortable if someone else can do it for you (Figure 4-33).

Cavity Press (Dian Xue, 點穴). There are six cavities that can be used to stimulate the Qi circulation deep in the neck: Fengfu (Gv-16) (風府), Yamen (Gv-15) (啞門), the two Fengchi (GB-20) (風池) cavities, and the two Tianzhu (B-10) (天柱) cavities (Figure 4-34). The thumb or index finger are most commonly used. When doing this on yourself, first concentrate your mind, and then gently press with a finger while keeping your neck relaxed. Press for three to five seconds and then let go. Five to ten presses are usually needed for proper stimulation. After doing the cavity press, place your attention deep inside the vertebrae and move your head around a few times.

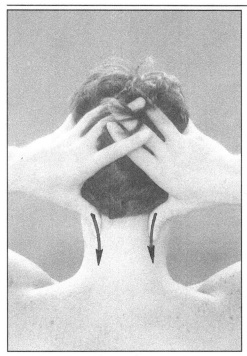

FIGURE 4-31

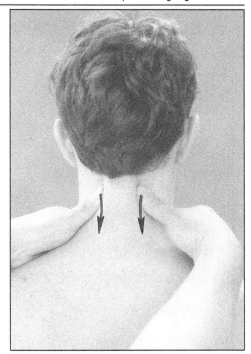

FIGURE 4-32

b. Spine 脊椎

Massage (An Mo, 按摩). Obviously, you need to have someone else massage your back. Before you can loosen up the spine, you must first loosen up the trunk muscles. Therefore, start at the neck and gradually work downward. Loosen the neck muscles as explained above, then grab and gently squeeze the muscles between the neck and the shoulders (Figure 4-35). This will help lead the Qi from the neck downward and spread it out across your back. Next, use the base of your palm (Figure 4-36) or the edge of your palm (Figure 4-37) to press the trunk muscles, moving down with a circular massaging motion. Massage from the neck down to the waist five to ten times. Do not massage upward, because this will lead the Qi in the wrong direction and cause stagnation.

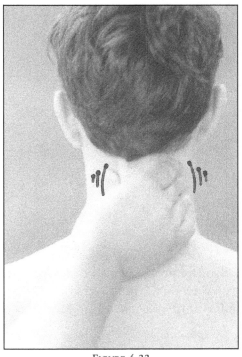

FIGURE 4-33

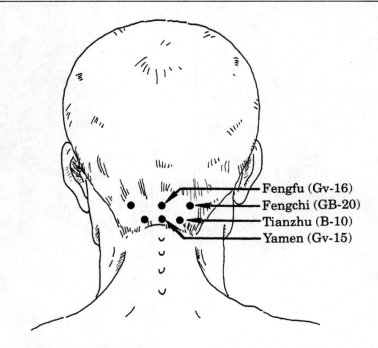

FIGURE 4-34. CAVITIES ON THE NECK

Fengfu (Gv-16)
Fengchi (GB-20)
Tianzhu (B-10)
Yamen (Gv-15)

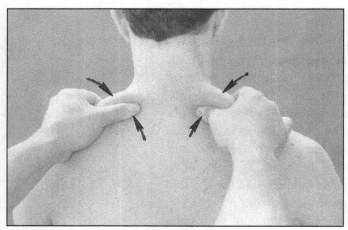

FIGURE 4-35

Once you have finished the circular pressing massage, place one hand on top of the other and press down on each joint in the spine. Do not press on the neck. Be sure that you press on the joints, and not on the vertebrae. The purpose is to bend and loosen the joints a little (Figure 4-38). Press in coordination with the patient's breathing.

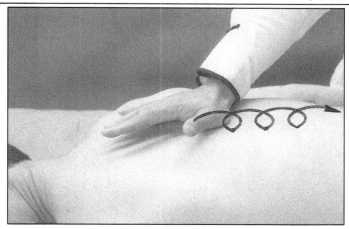

FIGURE 4-36

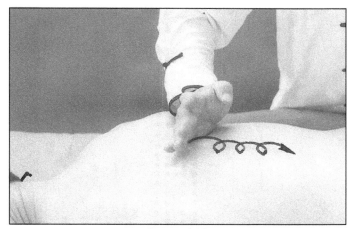

FIGURE 4-37

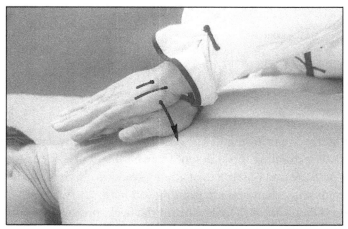

FIGURE 4-38

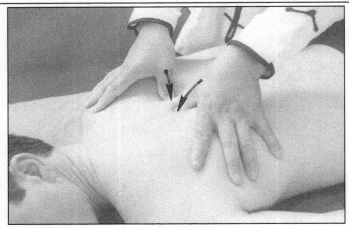

FIGURE 4-39

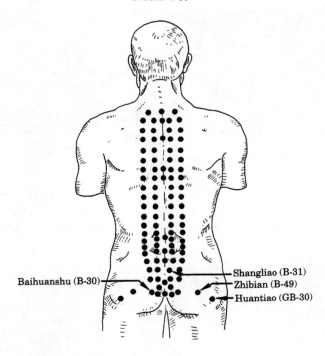

Baihuanshu (B-30)

Shangliao (B-31)
Zhibian (B-49)
Huantiao (GB-30)

FIGURE 4-40. CAVITIES ON THE SPINE

Place your hands in position and ask your patient to inhale deeply and then exhale. When your patient is exhaling, press down. How hard you press depends on the patient. Start with light pressure and observe the patient's reaction. If he or she holds their breath and tenses their muscles, then you are pressing too hard.

Cavity Press (Dian Xue, 點穴). Starting on the neck, press your thumbs into the gaps between the joints (Figure 4-39). When you have reached the tailbone, press the Shangliao

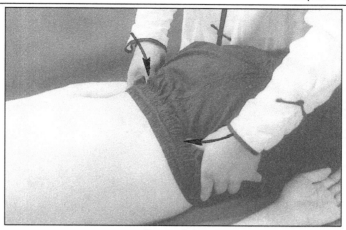

FIGURE 4-41

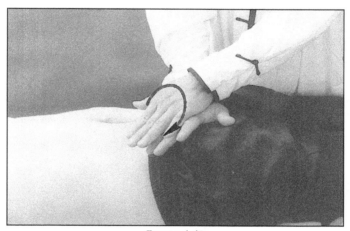

FIGURE 4-42

(B-31) (上髎), Baihuanshu (B-30) (白環俞), Zhibian (B-49) (秩邊), and Huantiao (GB-30) (環跳) cavities to lead the Qi to the hips (Figures 4-40 and 4-41). Finally, use the base of the palm to gently massage the sacrum for three minutes (Figure 4-42).

After you have finished pressing on the sides of the spine, repeat the procedure, only now press about two inches away from the spine. Figure 4-40 shows the cavities which should be pressed. After pressing, again use the palm to rub the trunk muscles, pushing to the sides and also downward (Figure 4-43). This procedure leads stagnant Qi sideways and downward away from the spine.

c. Waist 腰部

Massage (An Mo, 按摩). After you have massaged and loosened up the back, then start on the kidneys. Good Qi circulation in the kidneys is very important. When it is abnormal, the surrounding area will also be affected.

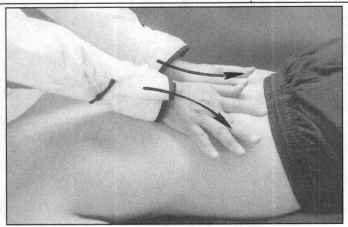

FIGURE 4-43

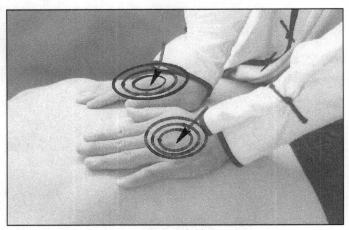

FIGURE 4-44

To massage the kidneys, use the same circular motion discussed earlier. It is best to have someone else massage your kidneys. If you are massaging someone, you may also press gently down on the kidneys with your palms, and then release the pressure (Figure 4-44). Do this about ten times and you will feel the release of tension in the kidneys and an improvement of the Qi circulation. Finally, use both palms to push from the kidneys to the sides of the body and also downward to the hips.

Next, press and release with your palms on the joint between the sacrum and the first vertebra about ten times (Figure 4-45), and then push to the sides and to the hips to lead the Qi there (Figure 4-46). An alternative way is to place your hands on the kidneys or waist and move your hands in circles. Keep your hands in contact with the skin so that they lightly brush it, but don't let them rub the skin (Figure 4-47). Use very little pressure, so that the patient is comfortable and doesn't feel any pain.

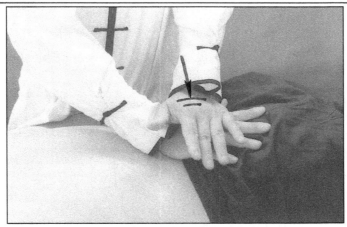

FIGURE 4-45

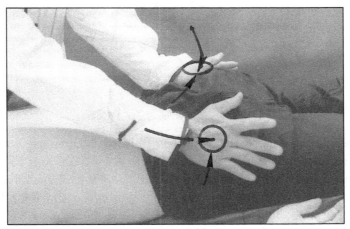

FIGURE 4-46

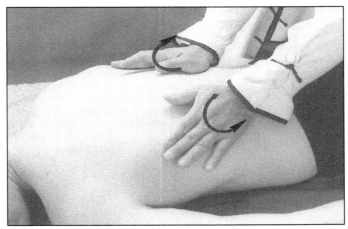

FIGURE 4-47

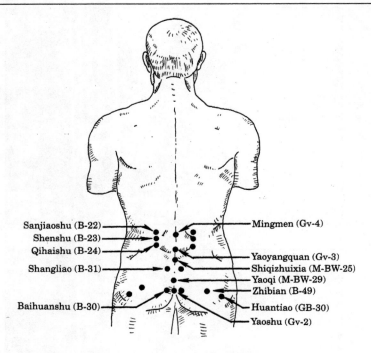

FIGURE 4-48. CAVITIES ON THE WAIST

Cavity Press (Dian Xue, 點穴). After you finished the massage, you can then use your thumbs to press the cavities shown in Figure 4-48. Start with Mingmen (Gv-4) (命門), and move down to Yaoyangquan (Gv-3) (腰陽關), Shiqizhuixia (M-BW-25) (十七椎下), Yaoqi (M-BW-29) (腰奇), and finally Yaoshu (Gv-2) (腰俞). Press each cavity three to five times, about three seconds each time. Next, press Sanjiaoshu (B-22) (三焦俞), Shenshu (B-23) (腎俞), Qihaishu (B-24) (氣海俞), Shangliao (B-31) (上髎), Baihuanshu (B-30) (白環俞), Zhibian (B-49) (秩邊), and Huantiao (GB-30) (環跳) cavities the same way to lead the Qi to the hips. Experience will teach you the appropriate pressing techniques and how to apply pressure. The more you practice, the more easily you will be able to penetrate with your pressure, and the more effective your cavity press will be.

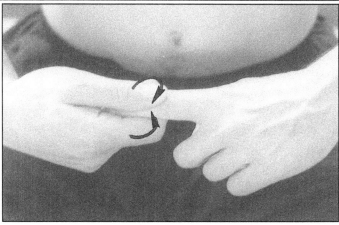
FIGURE 4-49

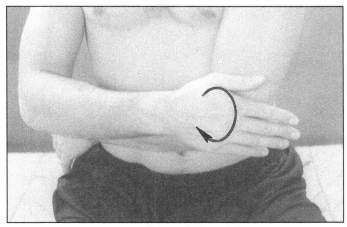
FIGURE 4-50

B. Joints in the Limbs 四肢關節

In this section, we will discuss a few of the techniques used for massaging the joints in the limbs. Once you are familiar with them, you may use the same theory to create others. Remember that the goal of massage is to loosen up the muscles and tendons and to increase the Qi circulation.

Massage (An Mo, 按摩)

Small joints such as in the fingers and toes can be held between the thumb and index finger while you apply circular pressure with the thumb (Figure 4-49). Move from one point to another until you have massaged the entire joint.

With the bigger joints—wrists, knees, elbows, and shoulders—place your palm over the joint and massage in a circular motion until the joint is warm (Figure 4-50). You can

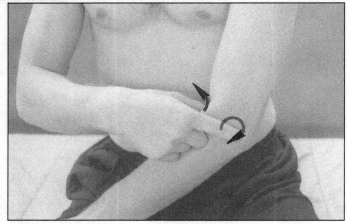

FIGURE 4-51

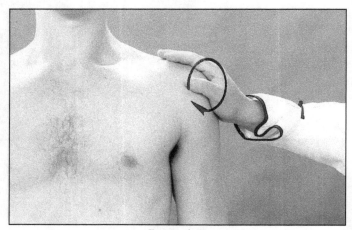

FIGURE 4-52

then press and circle in particular areas with a finger or thumb to stimulate the Qi circulation (Figure 4-51).

It is usually easier to have someone else massage your shoulder or hip. If you are the person massaging, use your palm (Figure 4-52), the edge of the palm (Figure 4-53), or the knuckles (Figure 4-54) to press in and rub. These are only a few of the many techniques that can be used to massage the joints and increase the Qi circulation.

As you practice you may discover many other ways to let your pressure penetrate deep into the joints.

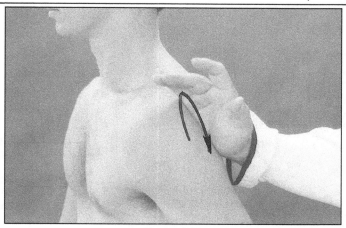

FIGURE 4-53

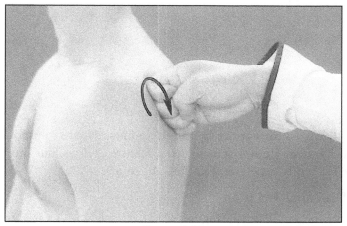

FIGURE 4-54

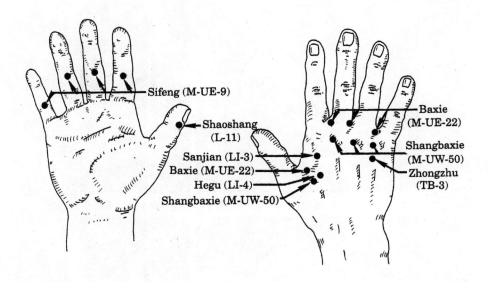

FIGURE 4-55. CAVITIES ON THE HAND

Next we will discuss the cavities or pressure points that are commonly used for cavity press. Some of them are not actually acupuncture cavities, but rather places where finger pressure can easily penetrate deep into the joints.

Cavity Press (Dian Xue, 點穴).

Hands (Fingers and Palms) (Figure 4-55). Hegu (LI-4) (合谷), Sanjian (LI-3) (三間), Baxie (M-UE-22) (八邪), Sifeng (M-UE-9) (四縫), Shangbaxie (M-UE-50) (上八邪), Shaoshang (L-11) (少商), Shaoze (SI-1) (少澤), Laogong (P-8) (勞宮), and Zhongzhu (TB-3) (中渚).

Wrists (Figure 4-56). Yangchi (TB-4) (陽池), Yanglao (SI-6) (養老), Yangxi (LI-5) (陽谿), Taiyuan (L-9) (太淵), Daling (P-7) (大陵), Shenmen (H-7) (神門), and Tongli (H-5) (通里).

Elbows (Figure 4-57). Quchi (LI-11) (曲池), Shousanli (LI-10) (手三里), Chize (L-5) (尺澤), Quze (P-3) (曲澤), Shaohai (H-3) (少海), and Xiaohai (SI-8) (小海).

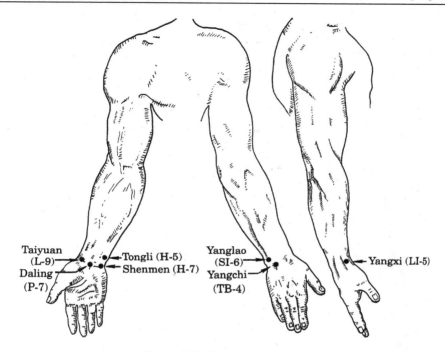

FIGURE 4-56. CAVITIES ON THE WRIST

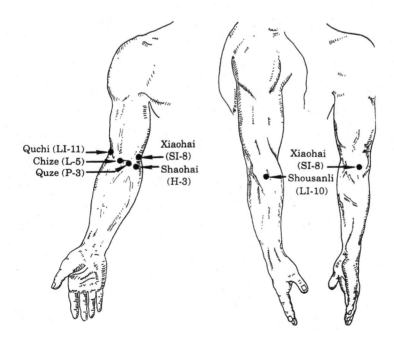

FIGURE 4-57. CAVITIES ON THE ELBOW

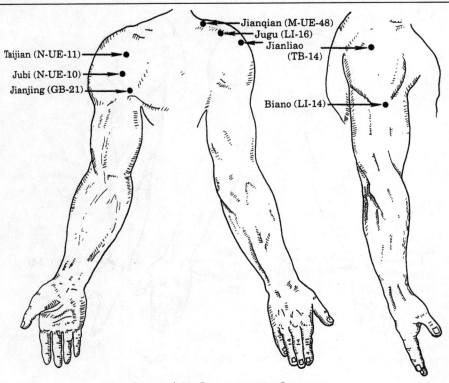

FIGURE 4-58. CAVITIES ON THE SHOULDER

Shoulders (Figure 4-58). Jianqian (M-UE-48) (肩前), Jugu (LI-16) (巨骨), Jianliao (TB-14) (肩髎), Jubi (N-UE-10) (舉臂), Taijian (N-UE-11) (抬肩), Binao (LI-14) (臂臑), and Jianjing (GB-21) (肩井).

Toes and Feet (Figure 4-59). Chongyang (S-42) (衝陽), Foot-Linqi (GB-41) (臨泣), Taichong (Li-3) (太衝), Xiangu (S-43) (陷谷), Zhiyin (B-67) (至陰), Bafeng (M-LE-8) (八風), Dadun (Li-1) (大敦), Yinbai (Sp-l) (隱白), and Yongquan (K-l) (湧泉).

Ankles (Figure 4-60). Jiexi (S-41) (解溪), Zhaohai (K-6) (照海), Taixi (K-3) (太谿), Kunlun (B-60) (崑崙), and Shenmai (B-62) (申脈).

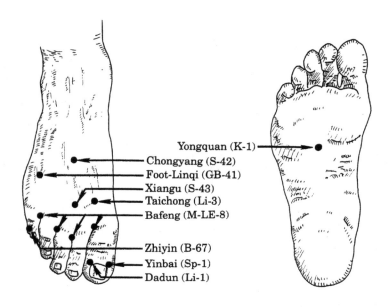

FIGURE 4-59. CAVITIES ON THE FOOT

Yongquan (K-1)

Chongyang (S-42)
Foot-Linqi (GB-41)
Xiangu (S-43)
Taichong (Li-3)
Bafeng (M-LE-8)
Zhiyin (B-67)
Yinbai (Sp-1)
Dadun (Li-1)

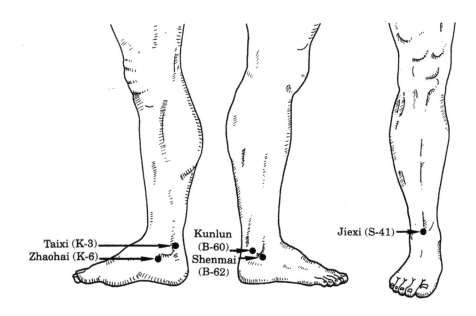

Taixi (K-3)
Zhaohai (K-6)
Kunlun (B-60)
Shenmai (B-62)
Jiexi (S-41)

FIGURE 4-60. CAVITIES ON THE ANKLE

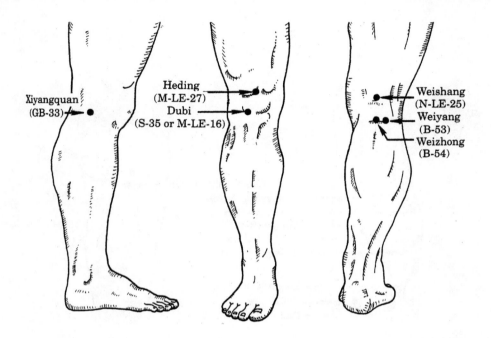

FIGURE 4-61. CAVITIES ON THE KNEE

Knees (Figure 4-61). Dubi (S-35 or M-LE-16) (犢鼻), Heding (M-LE-27) (鶴頂), Xiyangquan (GB-33) (膝陽關), Weizhong (B-54) (委中), Weiyang (B-53) (委陽), and Weishang (N-LE-25) (委上).

Hips (Figure 4-62). Femur-Juliao (GB-29) (居髎) and Huantiao (GB-30) (環跳).

4-4. QIGONG EXERCISES FOR ARTHRITIS 治療關節炎之氣功運動

Before introducing the Qigong exercises, we would first like to discuss the best time to practice Qigong. Experience indicates that the best time is in the early morning. The pain and stiffness of arthritis are most severe in the early morning because the Qi is most stagnant. If you can do some massage and some Qigong, you should be able to remove the stagnation and lessen the discomfort for the rest of the day. Therefore, in the early morning you should gently and lightly massage the joints until they are warm and the Qi circulation has increased, and then gradually and gently start the Qigong exercises.

You should also do the exercises right before you go to bed to smooth out any Qi stagnation. This will speed up the repair and healing of the joints while you sleep, and also lessen pain and stiffness the next morning. If you are able, you may add another practice session in the afternoon. Normally, your Qi is the strongest in the afternoon. You may take advantage of this to do Qigong exercises and lead Qi to the joints. Naturally, if you have the time, you may do the Qigong exercises whenever you can.

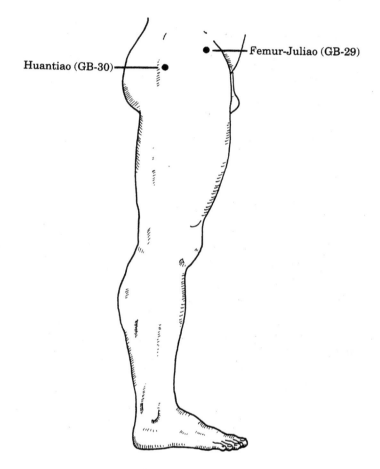

Huantiao (GB-30)

Femur-Juliao (GB-29)

FIGURE 4-62. CAVITIES ON THE HIP

There are a few things that you should be aware of. First, when the joint is inflamed you should not get involved in heavy Qigong exercise. Gently massage the joint to increase the Qi circulation, and then do some light and easy exercises. Second, when you have the least pain and stiffness, take advantage of the opportunity and practice a little more than usual. Third, do not overdo it. The way to judge this is that if about two hours after practice you still feel significant pain, then it was probably too much. The next time you should reduce the number of repetitions. With a little experience you will soon be able to judge what is right for you. Practice a comfortable length of time, and gradually increase the number of repetitions. Fourth, you should minimize the stress directly on the affected joints. As mentioned earlier, the best and most effective way is to bring the practice into your daily life and let it become a habit.

In this section, we will introduce a number of Qigong exercises which can be used to heal arthritis and rebuild the joints. Remember that the key to healing and regrowth is leading Qi to the joints and helping it to circulate smoothly there. The main way to do this is to concentrate your attention totally on the area you are exercising. When you concentrate, your Yi (mind) leads Qi to the joint. Breathing calmly and deeply also helps you to lead the Qi inward into the organs, joints, and bone marrow. Once you have grasped these tricks, you will be able to use the Qigong movements to circulate Qi in the joint smoothly and strongly.

When you practice, you should wear warm clothing and avoid exposing your joints to cold air or wind. After you practice, you should cover the joints and keep them warm. Remember that everyone is different, and you have to use your common sense to judge what is best for you.

When you are just starting these Qigong exercises, remember that you should not focus on building up the muscles and tendons. If you do this, your concentration will cause them to tense. This will increase the pressure in the joint and may cause the bones to grind against each other, which will hinder the healing process. Furthermore, although exercising the muscles and tendons may lead Qi to the joints, if you exercise too strenuously you will cause tension, which will stagnate the Qi circulation. You should always remember that *the key to good Qigong is using the mind and gentle movements to lead Qi to the joints and increase smooth Qi circulation.*

Once you have repaired some of the joint damage, you can then gradually start to emphasize strengthening the muscles and tendons. When the joints, muscles, and tendons are healthy, you have cured the arthritis. Remember that the strength of the joints must be built slowly and gradually. Do not expect to rebuild them in one night, one week, or even a month. However, after three months of consistent practice you should start to see improvement.

Qigong Exercises 氣功運動

A. The Trunk: 軀幹

Neck 頸部

The neck is the passageway to the brain for the Qi and blood. The brain is the center of your whole being, so if the circulation of the Qi and blood is stagnant or blocked, your brain will not receive the proper nourishment. This causes dizziness, headache, and in the long term, memory loss and accelerated aging. Blockages of the circulation to the head are often caused by neck injuries or arthritis in the neck joints. You can see that, in order to keep your brain functioning healthily, the first step is to remove any blockages of the circulation in the neck. The next two exercises are commonly used in China for this purpose.

Look Left and Right (Zuo Gu You Pan) 左顧右盼. This exercise can be done with the eyes open or closed, as long as you are able to concentrate your mind on your neck. Keep your mind calm, concentrate on what you are doing, and feel the movement of the

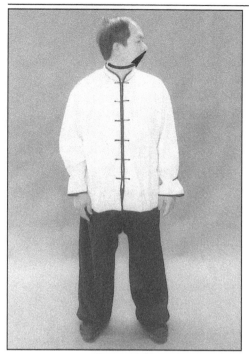

FIGURE 4-63

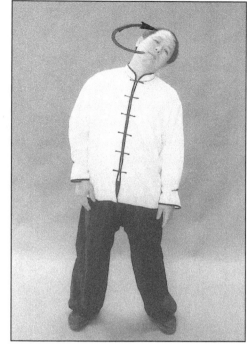

FIGURE 4-64

joints. The more you concentrate, the deeper you will lead the Qi.

The exercise is very simple. Simply turn your head slowly from one side to the other (Figure 4-63). You may sit or stand. As you turn your head to the side, exhale, and as you turn your head back to the front, inhale. Keep your neck as relaxed as possible. Keep turning your head until your neck starts getting warm, which may take twenty to fifty turns.

The Heaven Spins and the Earth Turns (Tian Xuan Di Zhuan) 天旋地轉. After you have finished the head turning exercise, continue by rotating your head. Remember, the circle should be small. Large circles may cause the neck vertebra to grind into each other, which will make the problem worse. Stay relaxed and concentrated. Simply rotate your head clockwise about twenty to fifty times and then counterclockwise another twenty to fifty times (Figure 4-64). Rotate your head the same number of times in both directions. When you have finished, close your eyes, keep your mind calm, and feel the Qi flowing in your neck area for a few minutes.

Spine 脊椎

According to Chinese medicine there is a Qi vessel called the Governing Vessel (Du Mai, 督脈) which follows the spine upward to the back of your head. Any problem with the spine can cause muscle tension, which, in turn, can cause stagnation of the Qi flow in the Governing Vessel. The Governing Vessel controls the six Yang primary Qi chan-

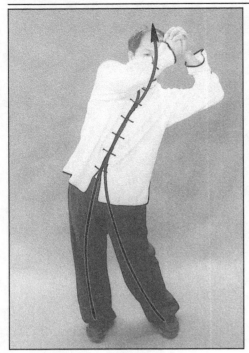

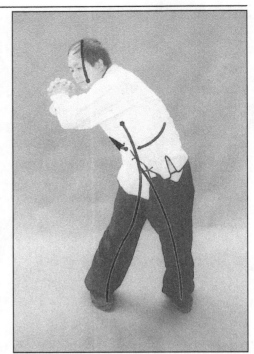

FIGURE 4-65   FIGURE 4-66

nels in the body (Large Intestine, Small Intestine, Triple Burner, Urinary Bladder, Gall Bladder, and Stomach channels). When there is any problem with the Qi circulation in the Governing Vessel, the six Yang primary channels and their related organs will also be affected.

Since any problem with your spine directly affects your health, Chinese Qigong pays much of attention to strengthening the spine and maintaining the Qi circulation in the back. The following movements are only some of the exercises that can be used to strengthen and maintain Qi circulation in the spine and back.

Large Dragon Softens Its Body (Da Long Ruan Shen) 大龍軟身. This exercise is a wave-like movement that starts at the legs and flows upward to the sacrum and finishes at the neck (Figure 4-65). The movement go from side to side and/or forward and backward. You may interlock your hands and move them along with your body. Keep your attention on your spine, where the movement is. You may also do this exercise sitting down, in which case you generate the movement in your abdomen and let it flow upward. The body remains as relaxed as possible. Practice from twenty to fifty times until the spine feels warm.

Large Dragon Turns Its Body (Da Long Zhuan Shen) 大龍轉身. Continue the wave movement described above, only now also start turning from side to side (Figure 4-66). The turning uses the trunk muscles to rotate the vertebrae, which increases the mobility of the spine.

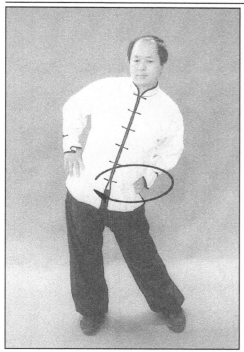

FIGURE 4-67

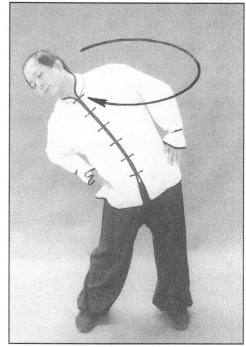

FIGURE 4-68

Waist 腰部

Be very careful when you exercise your waist. Moving too vigorously can injure the lower back and spine, so proceed slowly and carefully. The following three Qigong exercises can improve Qi circulation around the waist.

Rotating the Waist (Niu Yao Xian Huo) 扭腰現活. This is a very simple exercise. Keep your head and feet in place as you gently and smoothly move your waist in a circle (Figure 4-67). Circle ten to twenty times in one direction, and then repeat the same in the other direction. As you practice, pay attention to the waist area and try to feel the movement inside your body. When you can feel the movement of your spine, it means that you are leading Qi to it and at the same time using the motion to circulate it.

Lion Rotates its Head (Shi Zi Yao Tou) 獅子搖頭. In this exercise, keep your legs and waist in place and swing your upper body in a circle (Figure 4-68). You may also do this exercise while sitting on a chair. Move in one direction ten to twenty times, and then move in the reverse direction the same number of times. Remember to move gently. Your mind is always the key to success.

Bend and Straighten the Waist (Qian Gong Hou Ju) 前躬後鞠. This is one of the easiest Qigong exercises. In Chinese Wai Dan Qigong (外丹氣功), it is commonly used to massage the kidneys by tensing and relaxing the back muscles. It is also used to clear up waist problems and lower back pain. To do this exercise, simply relax your body as much as possible and bend forward. Swing your hips from side to side. Stay bent over for about five seconds and then gently straighten up (Figure 4-69). Repeat ten to twenty times. Once your waist has regained its strength, you may increase the number of repetitions. As always, keep your mind on the area being exercised.

B. Limbs 四肢

Arms

Hands (Fingers and Palms) 手

Usually when you exercise your fingers, your palms are also involved. In addition, since they are all connected, whenever you exercise your hands you are also to some degree exercising your wrists.

Chinese physicians have found that people who use their hands and fingers a lot are sick less often than people who don't. The reason for this is very simple. There are six

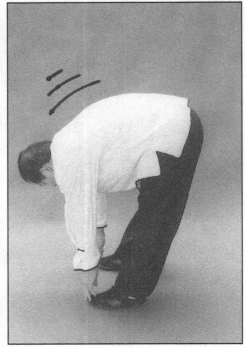

FIGURE 4-69

primary Qi channels that connect the fingers to six of your internal organs. Whenever you work with your hands, you build up Qi in those channels, and this Qi then flows into and nourishes the internal organs. There are many Qigong exercises for the hands. We will present four of them.

Swimming Octopus (Zhang Yu You Shui) 章魚游水 . This exercise also includes the wrists. Stretch your hands forward while spreading out the fingers (Figure 4-70), and then draw your wrists back while closing the fingers (Figure 4-71). Move your hands in and out, opening and closing the hands so that they look like a swimming octopus. If you wish, you may practice this one hand at a time. After doing this movement thirty to fifty times, your fingers, palms, and wrists will usually feel very warm. Remember, when you practice your hands should remain as relaxed as possible, and your mind should be concentrated on them.

Flying Finger Waves Gong (Zhi Bo Xiang Gong) 指波翔功 . This exercise is used by the Crane style of Gongfu to strengthen the palms and the base of the fingers. Simply bend your thumbs and fingers one after the other and then straighten them one at a time, repeating the motion in a sort of wave (Figure 4-72). Only bend the knuckles closest to the hands. If you bend the other knuckles you will fail to develop the base of the fingers. After you have done twenty to fifty repetitions, your palms and the base of your fingers should feel very warm and perhaps a little sore. After practicing, relax your arms as much as possible to allow the Qi that has accumulated in your hands to circulate to your arms and body.

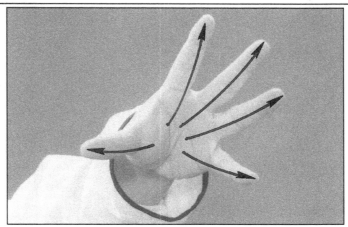

FIGURE 4-70

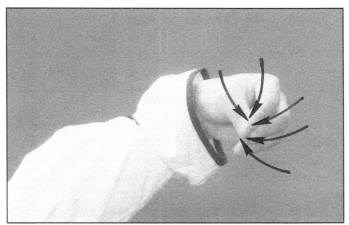

FIGURE 4-71

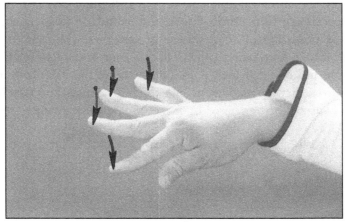

FIGURE 4-72

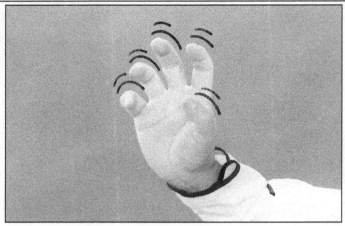

Figure 4-73

Tiger Claw Training (Hu Zhua Xing Gong) 虎爪行功. This exercise originated with the Tiger Claw style of Gongfu, and is more strenuous than the previous ones. This means that you should be more careful about how much tension you generate during practice. If your arthritis is very serious, you should probably not tense your muscles until your condition has improved, and then you should increase the tension very gradually.

To do this exercise, hold your hands like a tiger's paws (Figure 4-73) and gradually pull all of your fingers in to the center of the palms (Figure 4-74), and then open your hands again to the tiger's paw shape. After twenty to fifty repetitions, your fingers and palms should be very warm. When finished, relax your arms and allow the Qi to flow freely upward into your body.

Rolling the Taiji Ball (Zhuan Taiji Qiu) 轉太極球. In China, Taiji balls are well-known for their role in curing many illnesses, such as irregular Qi circulation in the six primary channels, and also local problems such as arthritis. Many arthritis patients have used Taiji balls to cure arthritis in the fingers and palms and to strengthen their joints.

Martial Taiji practitioners do a variety of exercises with various sizes of balls. However, the balls used for treating arthritis in the hands and wrists usually have a diameter of about one and one-half inches. In ancient times the balls were made of wood. Nowadays, however, they are made of metal, which is stronger and lasts longer.

Metal Taiji balls can be purchased in most Chinese department stores or martial art supplies stores.

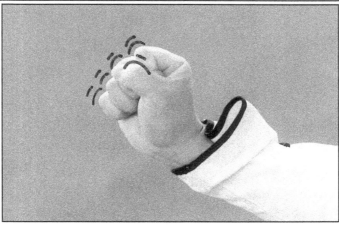

FIGURE 4-74

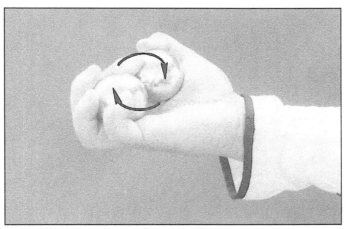

FIGURE 4-75

Taiji ball training for arthritis in the hands is very simple. Hold two of the balls in one hand and move them in a circle with your fingers to rotate them (Figure 4-75). Your hands should feel warm after only five to ten minutes. If you are patient and practice three or four times a day, you should see improvement in your arthritic condition in only a few months.

Once your arthritis has improved, you may start rebuilding the strength of your muscles by increasing the tension in your hands as you do the following exercises.

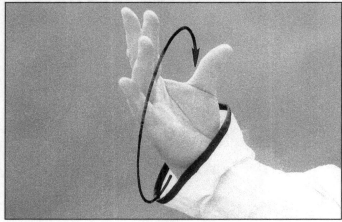

FIGURE 4-76

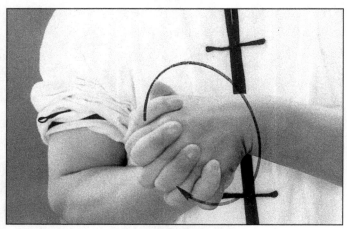

FIGURE 4-77

Wrists 手腕

Rotating the Wrists (Zhuan Wan) 轉腕. Rotating your wrists is very simple—you just relax your wrists and move your hands in circles (Figure 4-76). Keep your attention on your wrists to feel the rotation and make it as smooth as possible. Keep rotating until your wrists are warm, and then reverse the rotation and do the same number of repetitions. It usually takes 300 or more rotations before your wrists start to feel warm, especially in the wintertime.

Rotating the Wrists with Interlocked Fingers (Jiao Zhi Zhuan Wan) 交指轉腕. This exercise is similar to the previous one, only now the hands are interlocked and help each other. Lace your fingers together and move both hands in circles (Figure 4-77). Keep your attention on your wrists, and practice the same number of times in either direction. Once you have rebuilt your joints, this exercise can also be very helpful in rebuilding the tendons and muscles in your wrists. To do this, simply increase the tension on the wrists.

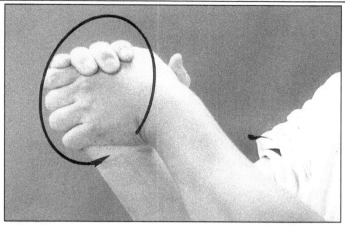

FIGURE 4-78

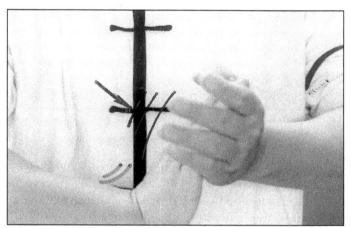

FIGURE 4-79

Rotating the Wrists while Holding Hands (Jiao Shou Zhuan Wan) 交手轉腕. This exercise is very similar to the previous one, only now, instead of interlocking your fingers, your hands are grasping each other (Figure 4-78). Again, keep your mind on your wrists and feel what is going on there. Once you have rebuilt the joints, you can increase the pressure to strengthen the tendons and muscles.

As you can see, the exercises are quite simple. You can easily discover other movements or exercises which lead Qi to the joints and increase their strength. For example, you can simply hold one hand steady and push it with the other one, and then relax. Push and relax until the wrist of the pushing hand starts to get warm (Figure 4-79).

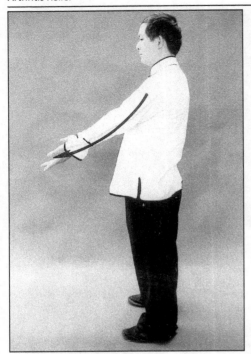

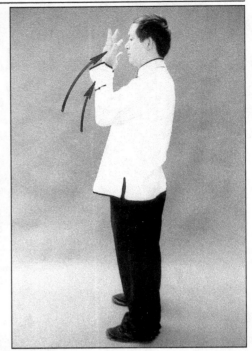

FIGURE 4-80   FIGURE 4-81

Elbows 肘

Lifting Movement (Shang Ti Wan Zhou) 上提彎肘. Extend your arms out in front of you with the palms up as if you were holding something (Figure 4-80). Raise your hands up to your face (Figure 4-81), and then lower them. Keep your mind on your elbows, and practice until they are warm. Then practice the same movement with the palms facing down. Once you are comfortable with this exercise, you can do it holding books or other light objects in your hands.

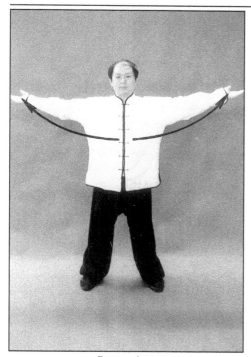

FIGURE 4-82

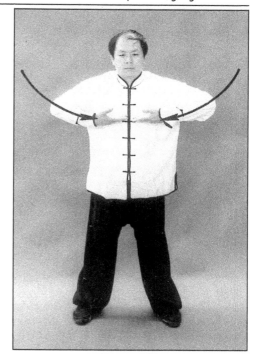

FIGURE 4-83

Sideward Movement (Nei Wai Wan Zhou) 內外彎肘. Extend your arms to the sides with the palms facing upward (Figure 4-82). Keeping your elbows in place, move your hands in to touch your chest (Figure 4-83) and then out again to the starting position. Keen your mind on your elbows and continue to practice until they are warm. Then turn your palms down and repeat the same movement. Once you are comfortable with the exercise, you can hold light objects in your hands as you practice.

Rotating the Elbows (Zhuan Zhou) 轉肘. Hold your arms in front of you as if you were driving a car. Keeping your elbows in place, move your hands in circles (Figure 4-84). Start with 50 repetitions of an inward motion, and then 50 times in the other direction. Don't make the circles too big, as this will put too much tension on the tendons in the elbows.

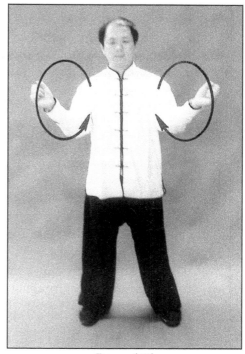

FIGURE 4-84

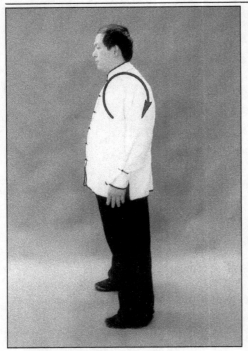

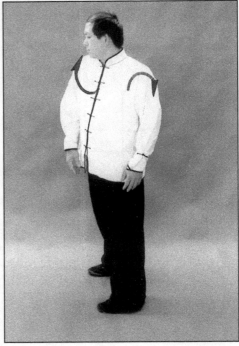

FIGURE 4-85 FIGURE 4-86

Shoulders 肩膀

Rotating the Shoulders (Song Jian) 鬆肩. Use your shoulder muscles to move both shoulder joints around. First circle forward about fifty times and then reverse the circling motion for another fifty times (Figure 4-85). Keep your mind on your shoulders, and keep them as relaxed as possible. Don't move too fast or you will cause muscle tension, which can hinder the Qi circulation.

You may also circle your shoulders with one of them 180 degrees behind the other (Figure 4-86). This motion has the advantage of moving your chest more, which increases the Qi circulation in the shoulders and helps any stagnant Qi there spread to the chest.

Front Waving (Qian Bo) 前波. This exercise comes from Crane martial Qigong. Move your arms like a crane's wings when it is flying. It is believed that cranes can fly long distances without rest because they know the key to circulating Qi in the joints where the wings connect to the body. Crane Gongfu emphasizes the shoulders in its Qigong training. This waving exercise is only one of many, but it is a key one in developing the Qi circulation and rebuilding the shoulder joints.

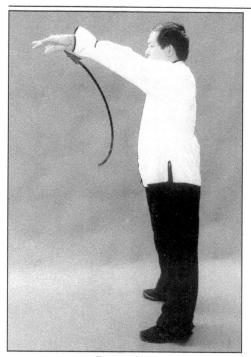

FIGURE 4-87

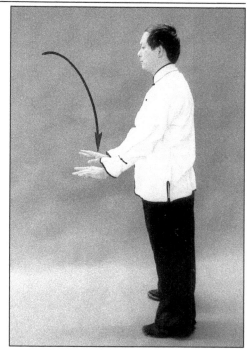

FIGURE 4-88

To do front waving, simply extend both arms in front of your chest and wave them up and down like flying wings (Figures 4-87 and 4-88). You may move both arms up and down simultaneously or one up and the other one down (Figure 4-89). The key to success is relaxing your shoulder joints as much as possible and moving your arms and chest together. If you can do this, the muscles and tendons in the shoulders will be very relaxed and the Qi circulation will be smooth.

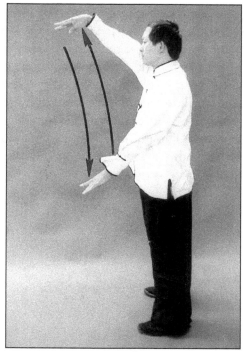

FIGURE 4-89

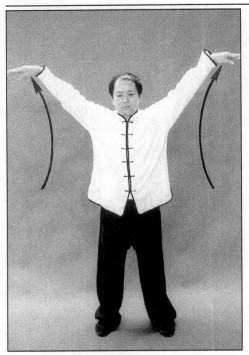
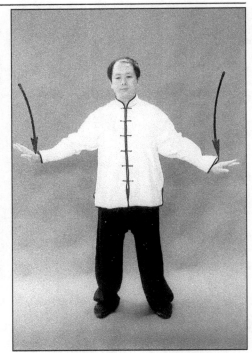

FIGURE 4-90   FIGURE 4-91

Crane Flying (He Xiang) 鶴翔 . Crane flying also comes from Crane style Qigong. This exercise is similar to the previous one, except now your wings (arms) are to your sides as they are on the bird. You may move both arms up and down at the same time (Figures 4-90 and 4-91), or move one up and the other one down. As in the previous form, treat your arms and chest as one unit and relax the shoulders to their maximum. You should fly until your arms are warm. If you train consistently, after a few months you will be able to increase the number of wing strokes to several hundred without feeling tired. This means that you will have rebuilt your shoulder joints. If you are interested in knowing more about soft White Crane Qigong, please refer to my book: *The Essence of Shaolin White Crane.*

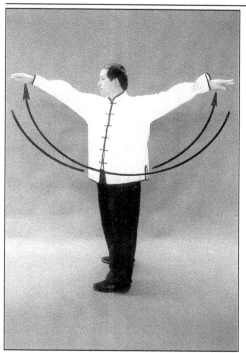

FIGURE 4-92

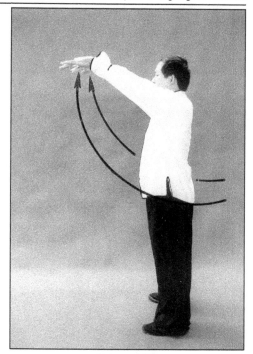

FIGURE 4-93

Front-Back Swinging Arms (Qian Hou Shuai Bi) 前後甩臂. This exercise is adopted from the way your hands swing while you are walking. Simply drop your arms naturally and comfortably beside your body (Figure 4-92), then swing one arm forward while the other swings backward. Turn your body from side to side and let your arms swing naturally. Swing them somewhat higher than you do when walking.

Alternatively, you may swing both arms forward and backward together (Figures 4-93 and 4-94). Arm-swinging Qigong has become very popular in Taiwan in the last twenty years since it has been proven to cure many kinds of illnesses, especially those related to the lungs and heart. Naturally, this exercise is also used for treating arthritis in the shoulders.

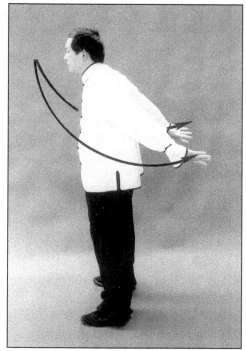

FIGURE 4-94

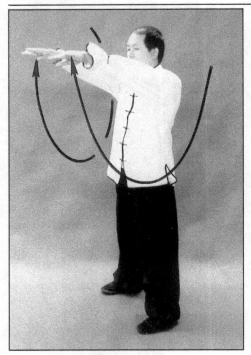

FIGURE 4-95

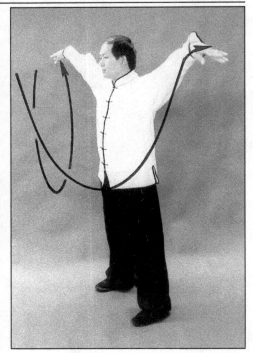

FIGURE 4-96

Front-Side Swing Arms (Qian Ce Shuai Bi) 前側甩臂. This exercise is very similar to the previous one, however, it comes from martial Crane Qigong. In this exercise you swing your arms in an undulating motion to the front and to the sides.

You may swing both arms forward and then sideward at the same time (Figures 4-95 and 4-96) or one forward and the other sideward (Figure 4-97). Extend your fingers but keep them relaxed. Keep your wrists relaxed too, so that they move slightly behind the arms.

After you have rebuilt your shoulder joints you may start to strengthen your muscles and tendons. You can do this by holding a weight in your hands while your are doing the exercises. Start with a light weight and gradually increase it.

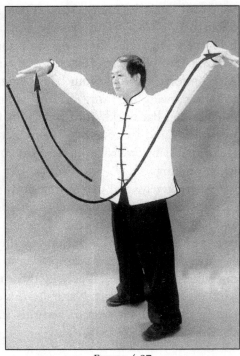

FIGURE 4-97

Legs

People in China know that walking is one of the most effective exercises for curing arthritis in the shoulders, hips, knees, and ankles. When you walk, your mind is peaceful and your body is relaxed. As you walk, pay attention to your stability, balance, and the motion of your joints. Swing your arms smoothly and lift your legs a little higher than usual. Start walking a mile or so, and increase the distance gradually as you get used to it. When the weather is too cold, or when it is raining, you can walk in place instead. When you feel comfortable walking, you can start walking uphill. On days when you can't go outside, you can walk up and down stairs. In China, when a patient has started walking again, physicians will frequently encourage him or her to walk up a hill in the morning, do some Qigong exercises, and then walk home.

In addition to walking, there are several other Qigong exercises that can be used to cure arthritis in the legs.

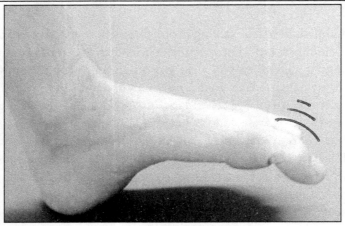

FIGURE 4-98

Toes 腳趾

Squeeze the Toes (Ji Jiao Zhi) 擠腳趾. Bend your toes down toward the centers of your soles and hold them there for about three seconds, and then relax (Figure 4-98). Keep your mind on the joints of the toes, and repeat the exercise until they are warm.

Up and Down Movements (Ding Zhi) 頂趾. Stand up on your toes for three to five seconds (Figure 4-99) and then lower yourself down onto your feet. This exercise is also very beneficial for arthritis in the ankles. Keep your mind on the joints of your toes, and repeat the exercise until they are warm.

Walking on the Toes (Zhi Xing) 趾行. This is the simplest exercise for the toes, feet, and ankles. Simply walk on your toes while paying attention to your feet (Figure 4-100). Walk slowly, keeping your body centered and balanced. After you walk about 100 steps, your feet will feel warm. You may then sit down and allow the Qi and blood to circulate upward. After you have rested for a while, you may repeat the exercise.

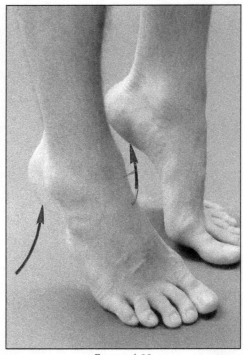

FIGURE 4-99

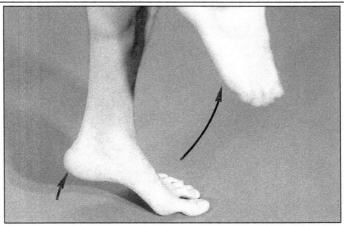

FIGURE 4-100

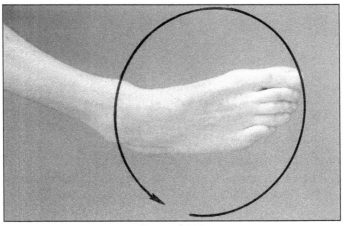

FIGURE 4-101

Ankles 踝關節

In addition to some of the toe exercises which are also beneficial for the ankles, there is another common Qigong exercise that can be used to improve the Qi and blood circulation in your ankles.

Rotating the Ankles (Zhuan Hua Guan Jie) 轉踝關節. If you are able, stand with your weight on one leg and move the ankle of the other leg in a circle. If you need to, you may use a wall or table for support. Circle in one direction 30 times and then reverse the direction and circle another 30 times (Figure 4-101). If you cannot do this exercise standing, you may do it sitting. Exercise slowly and pay attention to the movement of the joints so that you can feel the Qi moving there.

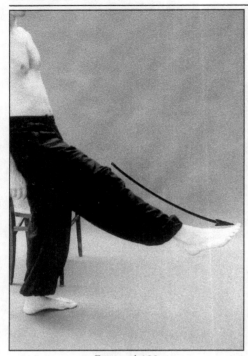

FIGURE 4-102

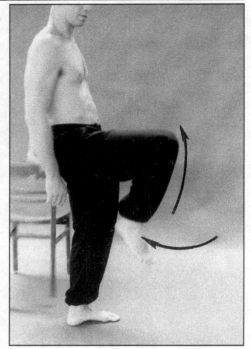

FIGURE 4-103

Knees 膝部

Straighten and Bend Movement (Wan Xi) 彎膝. When you do this exercise, you may stand on one leg or you may sit on the edge of a chair. Slowly straighten out your leg and then bend it (Figures 4-102 and 4-103). Repeat the exercise until the knee is warm, and then do the same number of repetitions with the other leg. Remember, it is your mind which leads the Qi to the joint, so keep your mind on the exercising joint and feel deeply into it. This way the Qi will be led deep into the joint. Once your knees are healthy again, you can start strengthening the muscles and tendons by placing a weight on your ankles as you exercise.

Moving the Body Up and Down (Xia Dun Shang Li) 下蹲上立. Simply bend your knees and squat down, and then stand up (Figures 4-104 and 4-105). When you start doing this, if your knees are too weak and give you too much pain, only bend them a little. Only when the strength of your knees has been rebuilt should you start squatting lower. Do the exercise slowly and keep your mind on your knees.

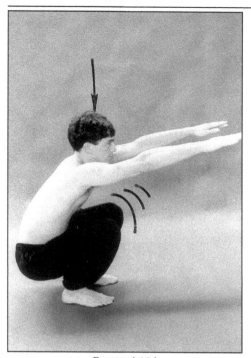

FIGURE 4-104

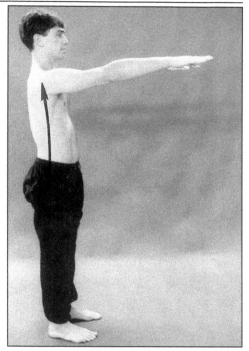

FIGURE 4-105

Horse Stance Training (Ma Bu) 馬步. Horse stance training is widely used in the Chinese martial arts to strengthen the knees. To do it, you simply squat down and stay there (Figure 4-106). Arthritis patients whose knees are not very strong should proceed very cautiously with this exercise. Only squat down slightly, and stay there for only 20 seconds or so. Once the knees are stronger, you can increase the length of time you stand, and also lower your body more to put more pressure on your knees. Horse stance training is one of the most effective techniques for rebuilding the muscles and tendons in the knees.

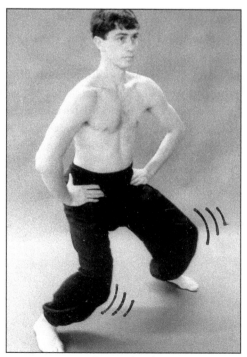

FIGURE 4-106

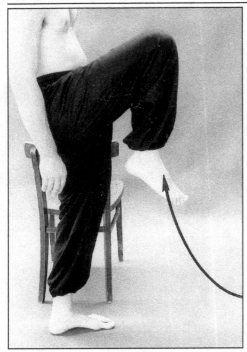

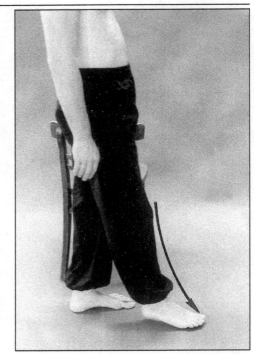

FIGURE 4-107   FIGURE 4-108

Hips 臀部

Raise and Lower the Leg (Shang Xia Ti Jiao) 上下提腳. If possible, stand on one leg, using a wall or table for support if necessary. Simply raise one leg and then lower it (Figures 4-107 and 4-108). Repeat 30 times and then change legs. Keep your mind on your hip joints and do the exercise slowly.

Sideward Motion and Rotating the Hip (Zuo You Zhuan Tun) 左右轉臀 you are able to lift your leg easily, move it to the side (Figure 4-109) and move it in a circle (Figure 4-110). Move slowly until the joints are strong again, and then increase the speed.

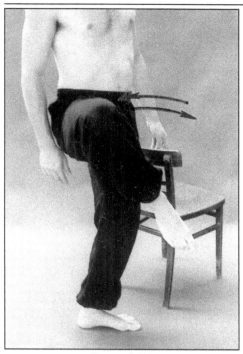

FIGURE 4-109

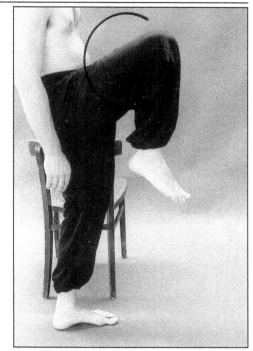

FIGURE 4-110

You can see that these Qigong exercises are not very different from the exercises you are already familiar with. What makes them different is that you are not just making a physical motion, you are also using your mind and attention to lead Qi to the joint to repair the damage and strengthen the muscles and tendons. You are also inhaling and exhaling deeply to move the Qi more efficiently into the joints and increase the Qi circulation. It is also important that you move slowly. This keeps the muscles and tendons relaxed, and allows the Qi to move more freely to the joint. When you move slowly it is also easier for you to keep your mind on the joint, and to feel deep inside it. Faster motions are harder to control, and can easily cause more damage.

CHAPTER 5

Conclusion 結論

When you practice Chinese Qigong, understanding the theory and principles is as important as the exercises themselves. If you understand the theory and principles, your mind will not doubt. Only when you feel confident about what you are doing will you continue to practice. Furthermore, if you understand the theory and principles, you can create variations or newer exercises that may suit you better and yield better results. It is not uncommon for people who do not understand the theory and principles to practice Qigong blindly and cause further injury. Therefore, when you practice Qigong, you should study and ponder its theory and principles.

Another thing you should realize is that no one can understand you, especially mentally, better than you can. The best way to heal yourself is to know yourself and understand the key to your individual problem. Then you can adapt the recommended methods to fit your particular problem and your personality. If you can do this, then the Qigong exercises which can benefit you will be naturally carried over into your lifestyle and become part of your life. This is the only way that you will continue to practice, and the only way that the benefits will really last.

As I mentioned in the beginning of this book, Chinese medicine has many ways or treating arthritis, and I know only a few of them. I hope that people who are qualified in other fields such as acupuncture and herbal treatment will contribute their knowledge and experience to fill this void.

In addition to introducing the West to the Qigong exercises for healing arthritis, I have had another goal in writing this book. I sincerely hope that this book will gain the attention of the Western medical establishment, and encourage them to become involved in Qigong experimentation, study, and research. This book is not an authority on this subject. It is, however, an attempt to open communication between East and West on the subject of medicine and healing. I deeply believe that if all of the different cultures can share their knowledge and experience and cooperate with each other, medical science will take a great step forward for the benefit of all humankind.

Translation and Glossary of Chinese Terms
中文術語之翻譯與解釋

Ai 哀 Sorrow.

Ai 愛 Love, kindness.

An Mo 按摩 Literally, press rub. Together they mean massage.

An Tian Le Ming 安天樂命 Means "be peace with Heaven and delight in your destiny." The typical attitude of scholar and Buddhist Qigong society.

An Yang, Henan province 河南、安陽 The location of an old Chinese capital during Shang Dynasty (1766-1154 B.C.) (商朝). It has become an important site for archeological study.

Ba Duan Jin 八段錦 Eight Pieces of Brocade. A Wai Dan Qigong (外丹氣功) practice that is said to have been created by Marshal Yue Fei (岳飛) during the Southern Song Dynasty (1127-1279 A.D.) (南宋).

Ba Kua (Bagua) 八卦 Literally, Eight Divinations. Also called the Eight Trigrams. In Chinese philosophy, the eight basic variations; shown in the Yi Jing (易經) as groups of single and broken lines.

Ba Kua Chang (Baguazhang) 八卦掌 Eight Trigrams Palm. One of the internal Qigong martial styles, believed to have been created by Dong, Hai-Chuan (董海川) between 1866 and 1880 A.D.

Ba Mai 八脈 Referred to as the eight extraordinary vessels. These eight vessels are considered to be Qi reservoirs, that regulate the Qi status in the primary Qi channels.

Bafeng (M-LE-8) 八風 Eight winds. The name of eight acupuncture cavities that belong to the Miscellaneous Points.

Bagua (Ba Kua) 八卦 Literally, "Eight Divinations." Also called the Eight Trigrams. In Chinese philosophy, the eight basic variations; shown in the Yi Jing (易經) as groups of single and broken lines.

Bai He 白鶴 Means "White Crane." One of the Chinese southern martial styles.

Baihuanshu (B-30) 白環俞 White circle's hollow. The name of an acupuncture point that belongs to the Bladder Channel.

Bao Pu Zi 抱朴子 *Embrace Simplicity.* Name of a well known Qigong and Chinese medical book written by Ge Hong (葛洪) during the Jin Dynasty in the 3rd century A.D. (晉朝).

Bao Shen Mi Yao 保身祕要 *The Secret Important Document of Body Protection.* A Qigong and medical book that describes moving and stationary Qigong practices, by Cao, Yuan-Bai (曹元白) during Qing Dynasty (1644-1911 A.D.) (清朝).

Baxie (M-UE-22) 八邪 Eight evils. The name of eight acupuncture cavities that belong to the Miscellaneous Points.

Bian Que 扁鵲 A well known physician who wrote the book, *Nan Jing* (*Classic on Disorders*) (難經) during the Chinese Qin and Han Dynasties (221 B.C.-220 A.D.) (秦,漢).

Bian Shi 砭石 Stone probes which were used to press the acupuncture cavities for healing before metal needles were available.

Binao (LI-14) 臂臑 Arm and scapula. The name of an acupuncture cavity that belongs to the Large Intestine Channel.

Cao, Yuan-Bai 曹元白 A well known physician and Qigong master who wrote a book called *Bao Shen Mi Yao* (*The Secret Important Document of Body Protection*) (保身祕要) that describes moving and stationary Qigong practices during the Qing Dynasty (1644-1911 A.D.) (清朝).

Chan (Ren) 禪,忍 A Chinese school of Mahayana Buddhism which asserts that enlightenment can be attained through meditation, self-contemplation and intuition, rather than through study of scripture. Chan is called Ren (忍) in Japan.

Chang 長 Long.

Chang Chuan (Changquan) 長拳 Means "Long Range Fist." Chang Chuan includes all northern Chinese long-range martial styles. Chang Chuan has also been used to refer to Taijiquan.

Changqiang (Gv-1) 長強 Long strength. The name of an acupuncture cavity that belongs to the Governing Vessel.

Changquan (Chang Chuan) 長拳 Means "Long Range Fist." Changquan includes all northern Chinese long-range martial styles. Chang Chuan has also been used to refer to Taijiquan.

Chao, Yuan-Fang 巢元方 A well-known physician and Qigong master during the Sui and Tang Dynasties (581-907 A.D.) (隋,唐). Chao, Yuan-Fang compiled the *Zhu Bing Yuan Hou Lun* (*Thesis on the Origins and Symptoms of Various Diseases*) (諸病源候論), that is a veritable encyclopedia of Qigong methods, listing 260 different ways of increasing the Qi flow.

Chen, Ji-Ru 陳繼儒 A well known physician and Qigong master who wrote the book, *Yang Shen Fu Yu* (*Brief Introduction to Nourishing the Body*) (養身膚語) about the three treasures: Jing (精) (essence), Qi (氣) (internal energy), and Shen (神) (spirit) during Qing Dynasty (1644-1911 A.D.) (清朝).

Cheng, Gin-Gsao (1911-1976 A.D.) 曾金灶 Dr. Yang, Jwing-Ming's White Crane master.

Chi (Qi) 氣 The energy pervading the universe, including the energy circulating in the human body.

Chi Kung (Qigong) 氣功 The Gongfu (功夫) of Qi, which means the study of Qi.

Chin Na (Qin Na) 擒拿 Literally means "grab control." A component of Chinese martial arts that emphasizes grabbing techniques, to control your opponent's joints, in conjunction with attacking certain acupuncture cavities.

Chize (L-5) 尺澤 Cubit march. The name of an acupuncture cavity that belongs to the Lung Channel.

Chong Mai 衝脈 Thrusting Vessel. One of the eight extraordinary Qi vessels.

Chongyang (S-42) 衝陽 Pouring Yang. The name of an acupuncture cavity that belongs to the Stomach Channel.

Chun Qiu Zhan Guo (770-221 B.C.,) 春秋戰國 The Spring and Autumn and Warring States Periods in Chinese history.

Da Mo 達摩 The Indian Buddhist monk who is credited with creating the Yi Jin Jing and Xi Sui Jing (易筋經；洗髓經) while at the Shaolin monastery. His last name was Sardili (剎地利) and he was also known as Bodhidarma. He was once the prince of a small tribe in southern India.

Da Zhou Tian 大周天 Literally, "Grand Cycle Heaven." Usually translated Grand Circulation. After a Nei Dan Qigong (內丹氣功) practitioner completes Small Circulation (Xiao Zhou Tian, 小周天), he will circulate his Qi through the entire body or exchange the Qi with nature.

Dadun (Li-1) 大敦 Great honesty. The name of an acupuncture cavity that belongs to the Liver Channel.

Dai Mai 帶脈 Girdle (or Belt) Vessel. One of the eight Qi vessels.

Daling (P-7) 大陵 Big tomb. The name of an acupuncture cavity that belongs to the Pericardium Channel.

Dan 丹 Elixir. In Qigong society, usually it implies the Qi circulating in the body that maintains the health and increases the longevity of your life.

Dan Tian 丹田 Literally, Field of Elixir. Locations in the body that are able to store and generate Qi (elixir) in the body. The Upper, Middle, and Lower Dan Tian are located respectively between the eyebrows, at the solar plexus, and a few inches below the navel.

Dan Tian Qi 丹田氣 Usually, the Qi which is converted from Original Essence and is stored in the Lower Dan Tian. This Qi is considered "water Qi" and is able to calm the body. Also called Xian Tian Qi (先天氣) (Pre-Heaven Qi).

Dao 道 The "way," by implication the "natural way."

Dao De Jing 道德經 *Morality Classic* or *Classic on the Virtue of the Dao*, written by Lao Zi (老子) (604-531 B.C.).

Dao Jia 道家 The Dao family. Daoism. Created by Lao Zi (老子) during the Zhou Dynasty (1122-934 B.C.) (周朝). In the Han Dynasty (c. 58 A.D.) (漢朝), it was mixed with the Buddhism to become the Daoist religion (Dao Jiao, 道教).

Dao Jiao 道教 Dao religion created by Zhang, Dao-Ling (張道陵) who combined the traditional Daoist principles with Buddhism during the Chinese Han Dynasty.

Di 地 The Earth. Earth, Heaven (Tian, 天) and Man (Ren, 人) are the "Three Natural Powers" (San Cai, 三才).

Di Li Shi 地理師 Di Li means "geomancy" and Shi means "teacher." Therefore Di Li Shi is a teacher or master who analyzes geographic locations according to the formulas in the *Yi Jing* (*Book of Changes*) and the energy distributions in the Earth. Also called Feng Shui Shi (風水師).

Di Qi 地氣 The Qi or the energy of the planet Earth.

Dian 點 "To point" or "to press."

Dian Mai (Dim Mak) 點脈 Mai means "the blood vessel" (Xue Mai, 血脈) or "the Qi channel" (Qi Mai, 氣脈). Dian Mai means "to press the blood vessel or Qi channel."

Dian Qi 電氣 Dian (電) means "electricity" and so Dian Qi means "electrical energy" (electricity). In China, a word is often placed before "Qi" to identify the different kinds of energy.

Dian Xue 點穴 Dian (點) means "to point and exert pressure" and Xue (穴) means "the cavities." Dian Xue refers to those Qin Na (擒拿) techniques that specialize in attacking acupuncture cavities to immobilize or kill an opponent.

Dian Xue An Mo 點穴按摩 One of Chinese massage techniques in which the acupuncture cavities are stimulated through pressure. Dian Xue massage is also called acupressure and is the root of Japanese Shiatsu.

Dim Mak (Dian Mai) 點脈 Cantonese of "Dian Mai."

Dong Han Dynasty 東漢 East Han Dynasty. A Chinese Dynasty during the period 25-168 A.D.

Dong, Hai-Chuan 董海川 A well known Chinese internal martial artist who is credited as the creator of Baguazhang in the late Qing Dynasty (清朝) (1644-1911 A.D.).

Du Mai 督脈 Usually translated "Governing Vessel." One of the eight extraordinary vessels.

Dubi (S-35 or M-LE-16) 犢鼻 This cavity is called "eyes of knee" (Xiyan, 膝眼). It is on the Stomach Channel and is also called "calf's nose" (Dubi, 犢鼻) when classified as one of the Miscellaneous Points.

Emei 峨嵋 Name of a mountain in Sichuan Province (四川省), China.

Fan Tong Hu Xi 返童呼吸 Back to childhood breathing. A breathing training in Nei Dan Qigong (內丹氣功) through which the practitioner tries to regain control of the muscles in the lower abdomen. Also called "abdominal breathing."

Feng Shi 風濕 Literally, "wind moisture," often translated as "rheumatism" in Western society.

Feng Shui 風水 Literally, wind-water.

Feng Shui Shi 風水師 Literally, "wind water teacher." Teacher or master of geomancy. Geomancy is the art or science of analyzing the natural energy relationships in a location, especially the interrelationships between "wind" and "water," hence the name. Also called Di Li Shi (地理師).

Fengchi (GB-20) 風池 Pool of wind. The name of an acupuncture cavity that belongs to the Gall Bladder Channel.

Fengfu (Gv-16) 風府 Wind's dwelling. The name of an acupuncture cavity that belongs to the Governing Vessel.

Gao, Tao 高濤 Master Yang, Jwing-Ming's first Taijiquan Master.

Ge Hong 葛洪 A famous physician and Qigong master who wrote the book, *Bao Pu Zi* (*Embrace Simplicity*) (抱朴子) during the Jin Dynasty (晉朝) in the 3rd century A.D.

Ge Zhi Yu Lun 格致餘論 Chinese name of the book, *A Further Thesis of Complete Study.* A medical and Qigong thesis written by Zhu, Dan-Xi (朱丹溪) during the Chinese Song, Jin, and Yuan Dynasties (960-1368 A.D.) (宋，金，元).

Gong (Kung) 功 Energy or hard work.

Gongfu (Kung Fu) 功夫 Means "energy-time." Anything which will take time and energy to learn or to accomplish is called Gongfu.

Guan Jie Yan 關節炎 Literally, "joint inflammation," and means arthritis.

Gui Qi 鬼氣 The Qi residue of a dead person. It is believed by the Chinese Buddhists and Daoists that this Qi residue is a so-called ghost.

Guoshu 國術 Abbreviation of "Zhongguo Wushu" (中國武術), which means "Chinese Martial Techniques."

Han Dynasty 漢朝 A dynasty in Chinese history (206 B.C.-221 A.D.).

Han, Ching-Tang 韓慶堂 A well-known Chinese martial artist, especially in Taiwan in the last forty years. Master Han is also Dr. Yang, Jwing-Ming's Long Fist Grand Master.

He 和 Harmony or peace.

Heding (M-LE-27) 鶴頂 Crane's top. The name of an acupuncture cavity that belongs to the Miscellaneous Points.

Hegu (LI-4) 合谷 Adjoining valleys. The name of an acupuncture cavity that belongs to the Large Intestine Channel.

Hen 恨 Hate.

Hou Tian 後天氣 Post-Birth Qi. This Qi is converted from the Essence of food and air and is classified as Fire Qi (Huo Qi, 火氣) since it can make your body too Yang.

Hsing Yi Chuan (Xingyiquan) 形意拳 Literally, Shape-mind Fist. An internal style of Gongfu in which the mind or thinking determines the shape or movement of the body. Creation of the style is attributed to Marshal Yue Fei (岳飛).

Hu Bu Gong 虎步功 Tiger Step Gong. A style of Qigong training.

Hua Tuo 華佗 A well-known physician during the Chinese Jin Dynasty in the 3rd century A.D. (晉朝).

Huan 緩 Slow.

Huan Jing Bu Nao 還精補腦 Literally, "to return the Essence to nourish the brain." A Daoist Qigong training process wherein Qi which is converted from Essence is led to the brain to nourish it.

Huang Di (2690-2590 B.C.) 黃帝 Yellow Emperor.

Huantiao (GB-30) 環跳 Encircling leap. An acupuncture point that belongs to the Gall Bladder Primary Qi Channel.

Huo Long Gong 火龍功 Fire Dragon Gong. A style of Qigong training created by Taiyang martial stylists.

Huo Qi 活氣 Huo means "alive." Huo Qi is the Qi of a living person or animal.

Jia Dan Tian 假丹田 False Dan Tian. Daoists believe that the Lower Dan Tian located on the front side of abdomen is not the Real Dan Tian. The Real Dan Tian corresponds to the physical center of gravity. The False Dan Tian is called Qihai (氣海) (Qi ocean) in Chinese medicine.

Jia Gu Wen 甲骨文 Oracle-Bone Scripture. Earliest evidence of the Chinese use of the written word. Found on pieces of turtle shell and animal bone from the Shang Dynasty (1766-1154 B.C.) (商朝). Most of the information recorded was of a religious nature.

Jianjing (GB-21) 肩井 Shoulder well. The name of an acupuncture cavity that belongs to the Gall Bladder Primary Qi Channel.

Jianliao (TB-14) 肩髎 Shoulder seam. The name of an acupuncture cavity that belongs to the Triple Burner Channel.

Jianqian (M-UE-48) 肩前 Shoulder front. The name of an acupuncture cavity that belongs to the Miscellaneous Points. This cavity is also called "Jianneiling" (肩內陵) (shoulder's inner tomb).

Jiao Hua Gong 叫化功 Beggar Gong. A style of Qigong training.

Jiexi (S-41) 解溪 Release stream. The name of an acupuncture cavity that belongs to the Stomach Primary Qi Channel.

Jin 筋 Means "tendons."

Jin Dynasty 晉朝 A Chinese dynasty in the 3rd century A.D.

Jin Kui Yao Lue 金匱要略 A Chinese book named *Prescriptions from the Golden Chamber*, which discusses the use of breathing and acupuncture to maintain good Qi flow. This book was written by Zhang, Zhong-Jing (張仲景) during the Chinese Qin and Han Dynasties (221 B.C.-220 A.D.) (秦，漢).

Jin Zhong Zhao 金鐘罩 Literally, "golden bell cover." A higher level of Iron Shirt training.

Jin, Shao-Feng 金紹峰 Dr. Yang, Jwing-Ming's White Crane Grand Master.

Jing 精 Essence. The most refined part of anything.

Jing 靜 Calm and silent.

Jing 經 Channels. Sometimes translated "meridian." Refers to the twelve organ-related "rivers" that circulate Qi throughout the body.

Jing Zi 精子 Literally, "essence son." The most refined part of human essence. The sperm.

Jubi (N-UE-10) 舉臂 Raise arm. The name of an acupuncture cavity that belongs to the New Points.

Jugu (LI-16) 巨骨 Great bone. The name of an acupuncture cavity that belongs to the Large Intestine Channel.

Juliao (GB-29) 居髎 Stationary seam. The name of an acupuncture cavity that belongs to the Gall Bladder Primary Qi Channel.

Jun Qing 君倩 A Daoist and Chinese doctor during the Chinese Jin Dynasty (265-420 A.D.) (晉朝). Jun Qing is credited as the creator of the Five Animal Sports Qigong (Wu Qin Xi, 五禽戲) practice.

Kan 坎 One of the Eight Trigrams.

Kong Qi 空氣 Space energy and implies air.

Kong Zi 孔子 Confucius. A Chinese scholar, during the period of 551-479 B.C., whose philosophy has significantly influenced Chinese culture.

Kun 坤 One of the Eight Trigrams.

Kung (Gong) 功 Means energy or hard work.

Kung Fu (Gongfu) 功夫 Literally, energy-time. Any study, learning, or practice that requires much patience, energy, and time to complete. Since practicing Chinese martial arts requires a great deal of time and energy, Chinese martial arts are commonly called Gongfu.

Kunlun (B-60) 昆崙 Kunlun mountains. The name of an acupuncture cavity that belongs to the Bladder Channel.

Kuoshu (Guoshu) 國術 Literally, national techniques. Another name for Chinese martial arts. First used by President Chiang, Kai-Shek (蔣介石) in 1928 at the founding of the Nanking Central Guoshu Institute.

Lan Shi Mi Cang 蘭室祕藏 *Secret Library of the Orchid Room*. Name of a Chinese medical and Qigong book written by Li Guo (李果) during the Song, Jin, and Yuan Dynasties (960-1368 A.D.) (宋，金，元).

Lao Zi 老子 The creator of Daoism, also called Li Er (李耳).

Laogong (P-8) 勞宮 Labor's palace. The name of an acupuncture cavity that belongs to the Pericardium Channel. The Laogong is located in the center of the palm.

Le 樂 Joy or happiness.

Li 離 A phase of the Bagua (八卦) (Eight Trigrams). Li represents fire.

Li Er 李耳 Nick-name of Lao Zi (老子). The creator of scholarly Daoism.

Li Guo 李果 A well-known Chinese physician and Qigong master who wrote the book, *Lan Shi Mi Cang* (*Secret Library of the Orchid Room*) (蘭室祕藏) during the period of Song, Jin, and Yuan Dynasties (960-1368 A.D.) (宋，金，元).

Li, Mao-Ching 李茂清 Dr. Yang, Jwing-Ming's Long Fist Master.

Lian 練 Means "to drill" or "to practice" to make stronger.

Lian Jing Hua Qi 練精化氣 To refine the Essence and convert it into Qi. One of the Qigong training processes through which you convert Essence into Qi.

Lian Qi 練氣 Lian means "to train, to strengthen and to refine." A Daoist training process through which your Qi grows stronger and more abundant.

Lian Qi Hua Shen 練氣化神 To refine the Qi to nourish the spirit. Part of the Qigong training process in which you learn how to lead Qi to the head to nourish the brain and Shen (spirit).

Liang Dynasty 梁朝 A dynasty in Chinese history (502-557 A.D.)

Ling Shu 靈樞 A well-known Chinese physician who wrote a medical book called: *Huang Di Nei Jing Su Wen* (*The Yellow Emperor's Inner Classic*) (黃帝內經素問) during Han Dynasty (circa 100-300 B.C.) (漢朝).

Linqi (GB-41) 臨泣 Near tears. The name of an acupuncture cavity that belongs to the Gall Bladder Channel.

Luo 絡 The small Qi channels that branch out from the primary Qi channels and are connected to the skin and to the bone marrow.

Mai 脈 Means "vessel" or "Qi channel."

Mencius (372-289 B.C.) 孟子 A well-known scholar who followed the philosophy of Confucius during the Chinese Zhou Dynasty (909-255 B.C.) (周朝).

Mian 綿 Soft.

Ming Dynasty 明朝 A Chinese Dynasty during the period 1368 to 1644 A.D.

Mingmen (Gv-4) 命門 Life's door. The name of an acupuncture cavity that belongs to the Governing Vessel.

Nan Hua Jing 南華經 Name of a book written by the Daoist philosopher Zhuang Zi (莊子) around 300 B.C. This book describes the relationship between health and the breath.

Nan Jing 難經 *Classic on Disorders.* A medical book written by the famous physician Bian Que (扁鵲) during the Qin and Han Dynasties (221 B.C.-220 A.D.) (秦，漢). *Nan Jing* describes methods of using the breathing to increase Qi circulation.

Nei Dan 內丹 Literally, internal elixir. A form of Qigong in which Qi (the elixir) is built up in the body and spread out to the limbs.

Nei Gong Tu Shuo 內功圖說 *Illustrated Explanation of Nei Gong.* Name of a Qigong book written by Wang, Zu-Yuan (王祖源) during the Qing Dynasty (清朝). This book presents the Twelve Pieces of Brocade (Shi Er Duan Jin, 十二段錦) and explains the idea of combining both moving and stationary Qigong.

Nei Jing 內經 *Inner Classic.* Name of a Chinese medical book written during the reign of the Yellow Emperor (2690-2590 B.C.) (黃帝).

Nu 怒 Anger.

Ping 平 Peace and harmony.

Qi (Chi) 氣 The general definition of Qi is: universal energy, including heat, light, and electromagnetic energy. A narrower definition of Qi refers to the energy circulating in human or animal bodies. A current popular model is that the Qi circulating in the human body is bioelectric in nature.

Qi Hua Lun 氣化論 *Qi Variation Thesis.* An ancient treatise that discusses the variations of Qi in the universe.

Qi Huo 起火 To start the fire. In Qigong practice, when you start to build up Qi at the Lower Dan Tian.

Qi Qing Liu Yu 七情六慾 Seven emotions and six desires. The seven emotions are happiness, anger, sorrow, joy, love, hate and desire. The six desires are the six sensory pleasures associated with the eyes, nose, ears, tongue, body and mind.

Qi Shi 氣勢 Shi means the way something looks or feels. Therefore, the feeling of Qi as it expresses itself.

Qi-Xue 氣血 Literally, "Qi blood." According to Chinese medicine, Qi and blood cannot be separated in our body and so the two words are commonly used together.

Qian Jin Fang 千金方 *Thousand Gold Prescriptions.* Name of a book written by a well-known Chinese physician and Qigong master Sun, Si-Miao (孫思邈) during the Sui and Tang Dynasties (581-907 A.D.) (隋，唐).

Qigong (Chi Kung) 氣功 Gong (功) means Gongfu (lit. energy-time). Therefore, Qigong means study, research, and/or practices related to Qi.

Qihai (Co-6) 氣海 Sea of Qi. The name of an acupuncture cavity that belongs to the Conception Vessel.

Qihaishu (B-24) 氣海俞 Sea of Qi hollow. The name of an acupuncture cavity that belongs to the Bladder Channel.

Qin Dynasty 秦朝 A Chinese Dynasty during the period 255-206 B.C.

Qin Na (Chin Na) 擒拿 Literally means "grab control." A component of Chinese martial arts that emphasizes grabbing techniques to control your opponent's joints, in conjunction with attacking certain acupuncture cavities.

Qing Dynasty 清朝 A dynasty in Chinese history. The last Chinese dynasty (1644-1912 A.D.).

Quchi (LI-11) 曲池 Crooked pool. The name of an acupuncture cavity that belongs to the Large Intestine Channel.

Quze (P-3) 曲澤 Crooked marsh. The name of an acupuncture cavity that belongs to the Pericardium Channel.

Re Qi 熱氣 Re means warmth or heat. Generally, Re Qi is used to represent heat. It is used sometimes to imply that a person or animal is still alive since the body is warm.

Ren 人 Man or mankind.

Ren 仁 Humanity, kindness or benevolence.

Ren Mai 任脈 Conception Vessel. One of the Eight Extraordinary Vessels.

Ren Qi 人氣 Human Qi.

Ren Shi 人事 Literally, human relations. Human events, activities and relationships.

Ren Zong 仁宗 One of the Song emperors during the period 1023-1064 A.D.

Ren (Chan) 忍 (禪) Means "to endure." The Japanese name of Chan (禪).

Ru Jia 儒家 Literally, "Confucian family." Scholars following Confucian thoughts; Confucianists.

Ru Men Shi Shi 儒門視事 *The Confucian Point of View*. Name of a book written by Zhang, Zi-He (張子和) during the Song, Jin, and Yuan Dynasties (960-1368 A.D.) (宋，金，元).

San Bao 三寶 Three treasures. Essence (Jing, 精), energy (Qi, 氣) and spirit (Shen, 神). Also called San Yuan (三元) (three origins).

San Cai 三才 Three powers. Heaven, Earth and Man.

San Gong 散功 Literally, "energy dispersion." A state of premature degeneration of the muscles where the Qi cannot effectively energize them. It can be caused by earlier over-training.

San Yuan 三元 Three origins. Also called "San Bao" (三寶) (three treasures). Human Essence (Jing, 精), energy (Qi, 氣) and spirit (Shen, 神).

Sanjian (LI-3) 三間 Between three. The name of an acupuncture cavity that belongs to the Large Intestine Channel.

Sanjiaoshu (B-22) 三焦俞 Triple Burner's hollow. The name of an acupuncture cavity that belongs to the Bladder Channel.

Shang Ceng Qi 上層氣 Upper level Qi and means the air (Kong Qi, 空氣) taken to the lungs through the nose.

Shang Dan Tian 上丹田 Upper Dan Tian. Located at the third eye, it is the residence of the Shen (神) (spirit).

Shang Dynasty 商朝 A dynasty in Chinese history during the period 1766-1154 B.C.

Shangbaxie (M-UE-50) 上八邪 Upper eight evils. The name of an acupuncture cavity that belongs to the Miscellaneous Points.

Shangliao (B-31) 上髎 One of four cavities on each side of the sacrum that belongs to the Bladder Primary Qi Channel.

Shaohai (H-3) 少海 Lesser sea. The name of an acupuncture cavity that belongs to the Heart Channel.

Shaolin Temple 少林寺 A monastery located in Henan Province (河南省), China. The Shaolin Temple is well known because of its martial arts training.

Shaoshang (L-11) 少商 Lesser merchant. The name of an acupuncture cavity that belongs to the Lung Channel.

Shaoze (SI-1) 少澤 Lesser marsh. The name of an acupuncture cavity that belongs to the Small Intestine Channel.

Shen 神 Spirit. According to Chinese Qigong, the Shen resides at the Upper Dan Tian (Shang Dan Tian, 上丹田) (the third eye).

Shen 深 Deep.

Shen Xin Ping Heng 身心平衡 Body and heart (mind) balanced. This means a balance between the physical body and the mental body.

Sheng Tai 聖胎 Holy embryo. Another name for the spiritual embryo (Shen Tai, 神胎).

Shenmai (B-62) 申脈 Extending vessel. The name of an acupuncture cavity that belongs to the Bladder Channel.

Shenmen (H-7) 神門 Spirit's door. The name of an acupuncture cavity that belongs to the Heart Channel.

Shenshu (B-23) 腎俞 Kidney's hollow. The name of an acupuncture cavity that belongs to the Bladder Qi Channel.

Shi Er Jing 十二經 The Twelve Primary Qi Channels in Chinese medicine.

Shi Er Zhuang 十二庄 Twelve Postures. A style of Qigong practice created during the Chinese Qing Dynasty (清朝).

Shi Ji 史紀 *Historical Record.* Name of a book written in the Spring and Autumn and Warring States Periods (770-221 B.C.) (春秋戰國).

Shiqizhuixia (M-BW-25) 十七椎下 Below 17 vertebrae. The name of an acupuncture cavity that belongs to the Miscellaneous Points.

Shousanli (LI-10) 手三里 Arm's three measures. The name of an acupuncture cavity that belongs to the Large Intestine Channel.

Shui Qi 水氣 Water Qi, which implies the Qi converted from Original Essence (Yuan Jing, 元精).

Si Qi 死氣 Dead Qi. The Qi remaining in a dead body. Sometimes called "ghost Qi" (Gui Qi, 鬼氣).

Sifeng (M-UE-9) 四縫 Four seams. The name of an acupuncture cavity that belongs to the Miscellaneous Points.

Song Dynasty 宋朝 A dynasty in Chinese history (960-1279 A.D.).

Southern Song Dynasty 南宋 After the Song was conquered by the Jin (金) race from Mongolia, the Song people moved to the south and established another country, called Southern Song (1127-1279 A.D.).

Su Wen 素問 Name of a medical book. The complete name of the book is called *Huang Di Nei Jing Su Wen* (*The Yellow Emperor's Inner Classic*) (黃帝內經素問). This book was written by Ling Shu (靈樞) during the Chinese Han Dynasty (circa 300-100 B.C.) (漢朝).

Suan Ming Shi 算命師 Literally, "calculate life teacher." A fortune-teller who is able to calculate your future and destiny.

Sui Dynasty 隋 A dynasty in China during the period of 581-618 A.D.

Sui Qi 髓氣 Marrow Qi.

Sun, Si-Miao 孫思邈 A well-known Chinese physician and Qigong master who wrote the book, *Qian Jin Fang* (*Thousand Gold Prescriptions*) (千金方) during the Sui and Tang Dynasties (581-907 A.D.) (隋，唐).

Taichong (Li-3) 太衝 Great pouring. The name of an acupuncture cavity that belongs to the Liver Channel.

Taijian (N-UE-11) 抬肩 Lift shoulder. The name of an acupuncture cavity that belongs to the New Points.

Taijiquan (Tai Chi Chuan) 太極拳 A Chinese internal martial style that is based on the theory of Taiji（太極）(Grand Ultimate).

Taipei 台北 The capital city of Taiwan located in the north.

Taiwan 台灣 An island to the south-east of mainland China. Also known as "Formosa."

Taiwan University 台灣大學 A well-known university located in northern Taiwan.

Taixi (K-3) 太谿 Great creek, The name of an acupuncture cavity that belongs to the Kidney Channel.

Taiyang martial stylists 太陽宗 A school of Chinese martial arts that practices Huo Long Gong（火龍功）(Fire Dragon Gong) Qigong training.

Taiyuan (L-9) 太淵 Great abyss. The name of an acupuncture cavity that belongs to the Lung Channel.

Taizuquan 太祖拳 A style of Chinese external martial arts.

Tamkang 淡江 Name of a University in Taiwan.

Tamkang College Guoshu Club 淡江國術社 A Chinese martial arts club founded by Dr. Yang when he was studying in Tamkang College.

Tao, Hong-Jing 陶弘景 A well-known physician and Qigong master who compiled the book, *Yang Shen Yan Ming Lu* (*Records of Nourishing the Body and Extending Life*)（養身延命錄）during 420 to 581 A.D.

Tian 天 Heaven or sky. In ancient China, people believed that Heaven was the most powerful natural energy in this universe.

Tian Qi 天氣 Heaven Qi. It is now commonly used to mean the weather, since weather is governed by Heaven Qi.

Tian Shi 天時 Heavenly timing. The repeated natural cycles generated by the heavens such as: seasons, months, days and hours.

Tianzhu (B-10) 天柱 Heaven's pillar. The name of an acupuncture cavity that belongs to the Bladder Channel.

Tiao Qi 調氣 To regulate the Qi.

Tiao Shen 調身 To regulate the body.

Tiao Shen 調神 To regulate the spirit.

Tiao Xi 調息 To regulate the breathing.

Tiao Xin 調心 To regulate the emotional mind.

Tie Bu Shan 鐵布衫 Iron shirt. Gongfu training which toughens the body externally and internally.

Tie Sha Zhang 鐵砂掌 Literally, "iron sand palm." A special martial arts conditioning for the palms.

Tong Ren Yu Xue Zhen Jiu Tu 銅人俞穴鍼灸圖 *Illustration of the Brass Man Acupuncture and Moxibustion.* Name of an acupuncture book written by Dr. Wang, Wei-Yi（王唯一）during the Song Dynasty.

Tongli (H-5) 通里 Reaching the measure. The name of an acupuncture cavity that belongs to the Heart Channel.

Tui Na 推拿 Means "to push and grab." A category of Chinese massages for healing and injury treatment.

Wai 外 External.

Wai Dan 外丹 External elixir. External Qigong exercises in which a practitioner will build up the Qi in his limbs and then lead it into the center of the body for nourishment.

Wai Dan Chi Kung (Wai Dan Qigong) 外丹氣功
External Elixir Qigong. In Wai Dan Qigong, a practitioner will generate Qi to the limbs and then allow the Qi to flow inward to nourish the internal organs.

Wai Jia 外家 External family. Those martial schools that practice the external styles of Chinese martial arts.

Wai Tai Mi Yao 外台祕要 *The Extra Important Secret.* Name of a Chinese medical book written by Wang Tao (王燾) during the Sui and Tang Dynasties (581-907 A.D.) (隋，唐). This book describes the use of breathing and herbal therapies for disorders of Qi circulation.

Wang Tao 王燾 A well-known Chinese physician and Qigong master who wrote the book *Wai Tai Mi Yao* (*The Extra Important Secret*) (外台祕要) during the Sui and Tang Dynasties (581-907 A.D.) (隋，唐).

Wang, Fan-An 汪汎庵 A well-known Chinese physician who wrote the book *Yi Fan Ji Jie* (*The Total Introduction to Medical Prescriptions*) (醫方集介) during the Qing Dynasty.

Wang, Wei-Yi 王唯一 A well-known Chinese physician who wrote the book, *Tong Ren Yu Xue Zhen Jiu Tu* (*Illustration of the Brass Man Acupuncture and Moxibustion*) (銅人俞穴鍼灸圖) during Song Dynasty (宋朝).

Wang, Zu-Yuan 王祖源 A well-known Chinese physician who wrote the book, *Nei Gong Tu Shuo* (*Illustrated Explanation of Nei Gong*) (內功圖說) during the Qing Dynasty (清朝).

Wei Qi 衛氣 Protective Qi or Guardian Qi. The Qi at the surface of the body that generates a shield to protect the body from negative external influences such as colds.

Wei, Bo-Yang 魏伯陽 A well-known physician who wrote the book, *Zhou Yi Can Tong Qi* (*A Comparative Study of the Zhou (Dynasty) Book of Changes*) (周易參同契) during the Qin and Han Dynasties (221 B.C.-220 A.D.) (秦，漢).

Weishang (N-LE-25) 委上 Above the commission. The name of an acupuncture cavity that belongs to the New Points.

Weiyang (B-53) 委陽 Commission the Yang. The name of an acupuncture cavity that belongs to the Bladder Channel.

Weizhong (B-54) 委中 Commission the middle. The name of an acupuncture cavity that belongs to the Bladder Primary Qi Channel.

Wilson Chen 陳威佯 Dr. Yang, Jwing-Ming's friend.

Wu Nian Zhi Nian 無念之念 The thought of no thought.

Wu Qin Shi 五禽戲 Five Animal Sports. A set of medical Qigong practice created by Jun Qing (君倩) during Chinese Jin Dynasty (265-420 A.D.) (晉朝).

Wu Tiao 五調 Five regulating methods in Qigong practice that include: regulating the body, regulating the breathing, regulating the mind, regulating the Qi, and regulating the spirit.

Wudang Mountain 武當山 Located in Hubei Province (湖北) in China.

Wuji 無極 Means "no extremity."

Wuji Qigong 無極氣功 A style of Taiji Qigong practice.

Wushu 武術 Literally, martial techniques. A common name for the Chinese martial arts. Many other terms are used, including: Wuyi (武藝) (martial arts), Wugong (武功) (martial Gongfu), Guoshu (國術) (national techniques), and Gongfu (功夫) (energy-time). Because Wushu has been modified in mainland China over the past forty years into gymnastic martial performance, many traditional Chinese martial artist have given up this name in order to avoid confusing modern Wushu with traditional Wushu. Recently, mainland China has attempted to bring modern Wushu back toward its traditional training and practice.

Xi 細 Slender.

Xi 喜 Joy, delight, and happiness.

Xi Sui Gong 洗髓功 Gongfu for marrow and brain washing Qigong practice.

Xi Sui Jing 洗髓經 Literally, *Washing Marrow/Brain Classic*, usually translated *Marrow/Brain Washing Classic*. A Qigong training that specializes in leading Qi to the marrow to cleanse it or to the brain to nourish the spirit for enlightenment. It is believed that Xi Sui Jing training is the key to longevity and achieving spiritual enlightenment.

Xia Ceng Qi 下層氣 Lower Level Qi. Means the Qi (bioelectricity) stored in the Real Lower Dan Tian (Zhen Xia Dan Tian, 真下丹田) (i.e. Second Brain).

Xia Dan Tian 下丹田 Lower Dan Tian. Located in the lower abdomen, it is believed to be the residence of water Qi (Original Qi).

Xian Tian Qi 先天氣 Pre-Birth Qi or Pre-Heaven Qi. Also called Dan Tian Qi (丹田氣). The Qi that is converted from Original Essence and is stored in the Lower Tian. Considered to be "water Qi," it is able to calm the body.

Xiangu (S-43) 陷谷 Sinking valley. The name of an acupuncture cavity that belongs to the Stomach Channel.

Xiao 孝 Filial Piety.

Xiao Zhou Tian 小周天 Literally, small heavenly cycle. Also called Small Circulation. In Qigong, when you can use your mind to lead Qi through the Conception and Governing Vessels, you have completed Xiao Zhou Tian.

Xiaohai (SI-8) 小海 Small sea. The name of an acupuncture cavity that belongs to the Small Intestine Channel.

Xin 心 Means "heart." Xin means the mind generated from emotional disturbance.

Xin 信 Trust.

Xin Xi Xiang Yi 心息相依 "Heart (mind) and breathing (are) mutually dependent."

Xingyiquan (Hsing Yi Chuan) 形意拳 Literally, Shape-mind Fist. An internal style of Gongfu in which the mind or thinking determines the shape or movement of the body. Creation of the style attributed to Marshal Yue Fei.

Xinzhu Xian 新竹縣 Birthplace of Dr. Yang, Jwing-Ming in Taiwan.

Xiu 修 Means "to regulate, to cultivate, or to repair."

Xiu Qi 修氣 Cultivate the Qi. Cultivate implies to protect, maintain, and refine. A Buddhist Qigong training.

Xiu Shen Si Ming 修身俟命 Cultivate the body and await destiny. A typical attitude of scholar and Buddhist Qigong society.

Xiyangquan (GB-33) 膝陽關 Knee's Yang hinge. The name of an acupuncture cavity that belongs to the Gall Bladder Channel.

Yamen (Gv-15) 啞門 Door of muteness. The name of an acupuncture cavity that belongs to the Governing Vessel.

Yan 言 Talking or speaking.

Yang 陽 In Chinese philosophy, the active, positive, masculine polarity. In Chinese medicine, Yang means excessive, overactive, overheated. The Yang organs are the Gall Bladder, Small Intestine, Large Intestine, Stomach, Bladder, and Triple Burner.

Yang Shen Fu Yu 養生膚語 *Brief Introduction to Nourishing the Body.* Name of a book written by Chen, Ji-Ru (陳繼儒) during the Qing Dynasty (清朝).

Yang Shen Jue 養生訣 *Life Nourishing Secrets.* Name of a medical book written by Zhang, An-Dao (張安道) during the Song, Jin, and Yuan Dynasties (960-1368 A.D.) (宋,金,元).

Yang Shen Yan Ming Lu 養身延命錄 *Records of Nourishing the Body and Extending Life.* A Chinese medical book written by Dao, Hong-Jing (陶弘景) in the period 420 to 581 A.D.

Yang, Jwing-Ming 楊俊敏 Author of this book.

Yang, Xie-Jin 楊謝盡女士 Name of Dr. Yang, Jwing-Ming's mother.

Yangchi (TB-4) 陽池 Pool of Yang. The name of an acupuncture cavity that belongs to the Triple Burner Channel.

Yanglao (SI-6) 養老 Nourish the old. The name of an acupuncture cavity that belongs to the Small Intestine Channel.

Yangxi (LI-5) 陽谿 Yang creek. The name of an acupuncture cavity that belongs to the Large Intestine Channel.

Yaoqi (M-BW-29) 腰奇 Lower back's miscellany. The name of an acupuncture cavity that belongs to the Miscellaneous Points.

Yaoshu (Gv-2) 腰俞 Lower back's hollow. The name of an acupuncture cavity that belongs to the Governing Vessel.

Yaoyangquan (Gv-3) 腰陽關 Lumber Yang's hinge. The name of an acupuncture cavity that belongs to the Governing Vessel.

Yi 意 Mind. Specifically, the mind that is generated by clear thinking and judgment, and that is able to make you calm, peaceful, and wise.

Yi 義 Justice or righteousness.

Yi Fan Ji Jie 醫方集介 *The Total Introduction to Medical Prescriptions.* Name of a Chinese medical book written by Wang, Fan-An (汪汎庵) during the Qing Dynasty (清朝).

Yi Jin Jing 易筋經 Literally, changing muscle/tendon classic, usually called *The Muscle/Tendon Changing Classic.* Credited to Da Mo (達磨) around 550 A.D., this work discusses Wai Dan Qigong (外丹氣功) training for strengthening the physical body.

Yi Jing 易經 *Book of Changes.* A book of divination written during the Zhou Dynasty (1122-255 B.C.) (周朝).

Yi Lu Mai Fa 一路埋伏 A Long Fist middle-level sequence.

Yi Shou Dan Tian 意守丹田 Keep your Yi on your Lower Dan Tian. In Qigong training, you keep your mind at the Lower Dan Tian in order to build up Qi. When you are circulating your Qi, you always lead your Qi back to your Lower Dan Tian before you stop.

Yi Yi Yin Qi 以意引氣 Use your Yi (wisdom mind) to lead your Qi. A Qigong technique. Yi cannot be pushed, but it can be led. The is best done with the Yi.

Yin 陰 In Chinese philosophy, the passive, negative, feminine polarity. In Chinese medicine, Yin means deficient. The Yin organs are the Heart, Lungs, Liver, Kidneys, Spleen, and Pericardium.

Yin Xu 殷墟 An archeological dig site of a late Shang Dynasty (商朝) burial ground.

Yinbai (Sp-l) 隱白 Hidden white. The name of an acupuncture cavity that belongs to the Spleen Channel.

Ying Gong 硬功 Hard Gongfu. Any Chinese martial training that emphasizes physical strength and power.

Yongquan (K-1) 湧泉 Bubbling Well. Name of an acupuncture cavity belonging to the Kidney Primary Qi Channel.

You 悠 Long, far, meditative, continuous, slow and soft.

Yu 慾 Desire.

Yuan Jing 元精 Original Essence. The fundamental, original substance inherited from your parents, it is converted into Original Qi.

Yuan Qi 元氣 Original Qi. The Qi created from the Original Essence inherited from your parents.

Yue Fei 岳飛 A Chinese hero in the Southern Song Dynasty (1127-1279 A.D.) (宋朝). Said to have created Ba Duan Jin (八段錦), Xingyiquan (形意拳) and Yue's Ying Zhua (岳家鷹爪).

Yun 勻 Uniform or even.

Zhang, An-Dao 張安道 A well-known Chinese physician and Qigong master who wrote the book, *Yang Shen Jue (Life Nourishing Secrets)* (養生訣), during the Song, Jin, and Yuan Dynasties (960-1368 A.D.) (宋，金，元).

Zhang, Dao-Ling 張道陵 A Daoist who combined scholarly Daoism with Buddhist philosophies and created Religious Daoism (Dao Jiao, 道教) during the Chinese Eastern Han Dynasty (25-221 A.D.) (東漢).

Zhang, San-Feng 張三豐 Zhang, San-Feng is credited as the creator of Taijiquan during the Song Dynasty in China (960-1127 A.D.) (宋朝).

Zhang, Xiang-San 張詳三 A well-known Chinese martial artist in Taiwan.

Zhang, Zhong-Jing 張仲景 A well-known Chinese physician who wrote the book, *Jin Kui Yao Lue* (*Prescriptions from the Golden Chamber*) (金匱要略), during the Qin and Han Dynasties (221 B.C.-220 A.D.) (秦，漢).

Zhang, Zi-He 張子和 A well-known Chinese physician who wrote the book, *Ru Men Shi Shi* (*The Confucian Point of View*) (儒門視事), during the Song, Jin, and Yuan Dynasties (960-1368 A.D.) (宋，金，元).

Zhaohai (K-6) 照海 Shining sea. The name of an acupuncture cavity that belongs to the Kidney Channel.

Zhen Dan Tian 真丹田 The Real Dan Tian, which is located at the physical center of gravity.

Zheng Qi 正氣 Righteous Qi. When a person is righteous, it is said that he has righteous Qi which evil Qi (Xie Qi, 邪氣) cannot overcome.

Zhibian (B-49) 秩邊 An acupuncture cavity belonging to the Bladder Primary Qi Channel.

Zhiyin (B-67) 至陰 End of Yin. The name of an acupuncture cavity that belongs to the Bladder Channel.

Zhong 忠 Loyalty.

Zhong Dan Tian 中丹田 Middle Dan Tian. Located in the area of the solar plexus, it is the residence of fire Qi.

Zhongliao (B-33) 中髎 Middle seam. One of four cavities on each side of the sacrum that belongs to the Bladder Primary Qi Channel.

Zhongzhu (TB-3) 中渚 Middle island. The name of an acupuncture cavity that belongs to the Triple Burner Channel.

Zhou Dynasty 周朝 A Dynasty in China during period of 1122-934 B.C..

Zhou Yi Can Tong Qi 周易參同契 *A Comparative Study of the Zhou (Dynasty) Book of Changes.* Name of a medical and Qigong book written by Wei, Bo-Yang (魏伯陽) during the Qin and Han Dynasties (221 B.C.-220 A.D.) (秦，漢).

Zhu Bing Yuan Hou Lun 諸病源候論 *Thesis on the Origins and Symptoms of Various Diseases.* Name of a Chinese medical book written by Chao, Yuan-Fang (巢元方) during the Sui and Tang Dynasties (581-907 A.D.) (隋，唐).

Zhu, Dan-Xi 朱丹溪 A well-known Chinese physician who wrote the book, *Ge Zhi Yu Lun* (*A Further Thesis of Complete Study*) (格致餘論), during the Song, Jin, and Yuan Dynasties (960-1368 A.D.) (宋，金，元).

Zhuan Qi Zhi Rou 專氣致柔 Means "concentrate on Qi and achieve softness." A famous saying written in Lao Zi's Dao De Jing (道德經).

Zhuang Zhou 莊周 A contemporary of Mencius who advocated Daoism.

Zhuang Zi 莊子 Zhuang Zhou (莊周). A contemporary of Mencius who advocated Daoism. Zhuang Zi also means the works of Zhuang Zhou.

Index